# NEGOTIATING
# PHARMACEUTICAL
# UNCERTAINTY

# NEGOTIATING PHARMACEUTICAL UNCERTAINTY

**Women's Agency in a South African HIV Prevention Trial**

Eirik Saethre
and
Jonathan Stadler

Vanderbilt University Press
Nashville

This book is printed on acid-free paper.
Manufactured in the United States of America

Library of Congress Cataloging-in-Publication Data on file
LC control number  2016015311
LC classification number  HQ29 S25 2017
Dewey class number  306.70820968—dc23
LC record available at lccn.loc.gov/2016015311

ISBN 978-0-8265-2139-2 (hardcover)
ISBN 978-0-8265-2140-8 (paperback)
ISBN 978-0-8265-2141-5 (ebook)

# Contents

# Acknowledgments

oremost, we would like to thank the participants in the MDP301 trial, as well as the men and women of Soweto and Orange Farm. These people graciously and openly shared their outlooks, experiences, and aspirations with us. Without them, this book would not have been possible.

We must also acknowledge the contributions of the hundreds of people—clinicians, administrators, managers, nurses, and assistants—who worked tirelessly on the MDP301. We are especially grateful to our colleagues in Johannesburg at the Wits Reproductive Health and HIV Institute (WRHI), including Helen Rees, Sinead Delany-Moretlwe, Sibongile Walaza, Jocelyn Moyes, and Thesla Palanee-Phillips. At the MDP301 in London, Sheena McCormack, Charles Lacey, Robert Pool, and Catherine Montgomery supported our work, as did our social science colleagues from other MDP301 trial sites: Oliver Mweemba, Agnes Ssali, Mitzy Gafos, Shelley Lees, Andrew Vallely, Gita Ramjee, and Neetha Morar. We would also like to recognize the assistance of Johannesburg site staff and thank those with whom we worked closely on the social science research component: Mdu Mntambo, Sello Seoka, Florence Mathebula, Edmond Mudau, Thembakazi Mantshule, Elisa Shikwane, Neo Mohajane, and Zelda Masango.

Throughout the conceptualization and writing of this book, we have benefited enormously from the insights of and feedback from Isak Niehaus, John Sharp, Fraser McNeill, Jimmy Pieterse, Mary Crew, Robert Thornton, David Copland, and Catherine Burns.

Through the MDP301, our work has received significant financial support from the United Kingdom's Department for International Development (DFID) and the Medical Research Council. Additional funding was supplied by the International Partnership for Microbicides, the European and Developing Countries Clinical Trials Partnership, and the Wellcome Trust.

Eirik Saethre's research activities were additionally funded through a post-doctoral fellowship at the University of Pretoria. His travel to South Africa was financed through the generous support of the WRHI. Jonathan Stadler's work was additionally sponsored by UK Aid from the DFID through the STRIVE Research Programme Consortium.

# Introduction

As pharmaceuticals have come to revolutionize the treatment of diseases such as HIV, cancer, hypertension, and depression, drugs are being developed, tested, licensed, marketed, and consumed at an ever-increasing rate. Each year, scientists and doctors celebrate as new medicines emerge from clinical testing. However, for every pharmaceutical that is proven to work, many more are found to be ineffective. This is the story of an unsuccessful HIV prevention drug, the international clinical trial that tested it, and the thousands of African women who participated in the trial. Much more than a series of physical exams and statistical calculations, medical research powerfully reconfigures the lives of those involved, changing attitudes, expectations, and aspirations. While ostensibly a tale of pharmaceutical failure, this is also a tale of hope, biomedical ambiguity, and female agency.

From 2005 to 2009, the Microbicides Development Programme 301 (MDP301) was a large international clinical trial designed to test the efficacy of a new microbicide, PRO 2000/5. An innovative biotechnology, microbicides function by disabling viruses or preventing their entry into host cells. It is hoped that microbicides—suspended in gels, films, creams, or rings that are used vaginally—will one day provide a way of arresting HIV transmission without the use of condoms. Optimistic that PRO 2000/5 would be the first efficacious microbicide, the MDP301 enrolled 9,389 women at 6 sites: Zambia, Uganda, Tanzania, and 3 locations in South Africa. Although the trial was conducted solely within Africa, PRO 2000/5 was manufactured by a pharmaceutical company in the United States, while trial funding came from the British Medical Research Council. In 2009, after four years of testing, the trial reported that PRO 2000/5 was not harmful, but neither did it prevent HIV infection (McCormack et al. 2010). In short, PRO 2000/5 didn't work.

While the results might appear to be simple, the reactions to them and the trial itself were decidedly complex. Microbicide advocates and researchers were careful to note that the trial was not a failure, because it had objectively proved that the gel was harmless but also ineffective against HIV. As some trialists focused on the science of the MDP301, others evaluated its financial and social outcomes, saying that it had increased infrastructural and research resources in Africa as well as positively impacting trial participants. Although PRO 2000/5 did not prevent the spread of HIV, advocates stressed that the MDP301 had demonstrated that microbicides could improve the lives of African women. Sheena McCormack, the chair of the MDP301, declared that microbicide researchers had the "method right," recommending a redoubling of efforts to find an effective product (Citizen News Service 2009). Rather than being categorized as a total failure, the MDP301 was often portrayed as a qualified success.

Meanwhile, southern African government officials, journalists, and citizens had long questioned the ethics and outcomes of the clinical trials conducted on their continent. A few years prior to the MDP301, microbicide trials testing nonoxynol-9 and cellulose sulphate had put participants at higher risk for contracting HIV. Although PRO 2000/5 was found to be harmless, 123 participants on the placebo and 130 participants on the 0.5 percent arm did contract HIV while enrolled in the trial. Edwin Mapara, a London-based Zimbabwean medical doctor, responded to the results with strong words:

> This is simply sanctioned murder (Grievous Bodily Harm) FROM THE WEST, in the name of scientific research, by the Medical Research Council and DFID [Department for International Development] at a cost of £40 million to infect ONLY one hundred and twenty-three (123) simple, cheap, black, AFRICAN women's lives in Uganda, Tanzania, South Africa and Zambia. *The lead researcher says, "IT IS DISHEARTENING!"* No it is MURDER! (quoted in Tatoud 2012; emphasis in original)

For Mapara and others who shared his view, the MDP301 was not merely a failure, but an orchestrated exercise in infecting Africans with HIV. Equated with colonial exploitation, clinical trials like the MDP301 are increasingly seen as sinister, anti-African enterprises controlled by foreigners.

Although Mapara and McCormack differ on the outcome of the MDP301, they do agree that its participants were impoverished, vulnerable

African women, whom they portray as the victims of more powerful agents. Whether the MDP301 is viewed as a foreign exploitative enterprise or one designed to empower African women, its participants are cast as passive and unable to resist either the coercion of the trial or the agency of men. While critics of clinical trials underscore the helplessness of women, the voices of participants are conspicuously absent in these accounts, as they are in the trials themselves. Because trials strive to eliminate social bias through randomization, double-blinding, and careful physiological assessments, trial researchers consider the perceptions of participants largely irrelevant. But as anthropologists who have spent many years working in and around clinical trials, we believe that the experiences and beliefs of trial participants are critical. Examining relationships that are often overlooked, we seek to reframe scientific endeavors as social endeavors. By foregrounding the perspectives of women who enrolled in the MDP301 and shifting the focus from idealized models and homogenizing statistics to the complexities of participants' lives, we illustrate the profound impact that international medical research can have on the communities in which it is conducted.

Boikanyo was one of the many women whose lives were impacted by the MDP301. She was 22 years old at the time of her enrollment and lived in an informal settlement next to Soweto's Chris Hani Baragwanath Hospital. Although they are only a short drive from the wealthy malls of northern Johannesburg, townships like Soweto are characterized by high rates of poverty, unemployment, and crime. Like the overwhelming majority of MDP301 participants, Boikanyo was often unemployed and unable to support herself. She lived in a two-room shack with her mother and brother. Boikanyo had been in a relationship for about a year and commented that her boyfriend was "sweet" and never yelled at her or beat her, as boyfriends often did. Nevertheless, she felt vulnerable. Having already contracted genital herpes, Boikanyo worried that she would soon become infected with HIV. Although a few of her neighbors told her that the MDP301 would give her AIDS, Boikanyo discounted these rumors and joined the trial in part to gain access to regular HIV testing and health screening. But for Boikanyo and many other participants, the MDP301 was much more than a way to monitor health. Boikanyo said:

> I feel like I am making a difference in the world even though other people don't see it. I feel I am contributing in this world because people

are dying since there isn't a cure for AIDS. I have seen a lot of people die in front of me from AIDS. My aunt recently passed away from AIDS as well. That's why I feel as though I am making a difference even though other people are not able to see it. I know I can't change the whole world but by being a part of this study, I know that I have to use condoms and I have to use the [microbicide] gel so that I can stay HIV negative. By following study procedures and doing what I am supposed to do, then that is going to help me and protect me from dying at a young age and upsetting my mother. That's why I feel like I am making a difference.[1]

For Boikanyo, trial participation was intimately tied to memories of watching friends and family die of HIV. Furthermore, she saw trial enrollment as an opportunity to contribute in her own way to the health of millions of Africans. Echoing these remarks, women repeatedly told us that in risking their bodies for the well-being of others through trial participation, they had gained control of their lives. Far from being vulnerable, women portrayed themselves as powerful. Examining the experiences of Boikanyo and other participants such as Kagiso, Mandisa, Andiswa, Zinzi, Zanele, Precious, and Nomsa, the story of a failed pharmaceutical is transformed into one of hope, sacrifice, and salvation.

## PHARMACEUTICAL ASPIRATIONS IN THE AGE OF AIDS

Over the last few decades, AIDS went from a mysterious illness that appeared to be killing gay men in the United States to a global epidemic affecting tens of millions of people. Much more than a disease, AIDS embodies fear and hope. Illness and medicine have always been powerful lenses through which to examine the world (Briggs and Mantini-Briggs 2004; Crandon-Malamud 1993; Kleinman 1980) and AIDS is no exception. Social meanings are particularly evident in epidemics, which Fassin (2007:32) characterizes as "moments of truth when both knowledge and power are put to the test." Uncovering rather than inventing, epidemics create a space through which social beliefs and attitudes are laid bare. AIDS has been referred to as an "epidemic of signification," and its discourse has historically mimicked and reinforced popular stereotypes of gay men, women, and Africans (Treichler 1999). Yet the rise of AIDS advocacy and the push for universal access to HIV treatments have also succeeded in reconfiguring relationships between governments, pharmaceutical companies, and private citizens (Biehl 2009). As a result, the AIDS pandemic and the many interventions designed to counter it have "given birth to unfamiliar forms of sociality and signification, enterprise, and activism— both negative and positive" (Comaroff and Comaroff 2011:179). While AIDS discourse draws from long-standing conversations regarding gender, sexuality, and illness, it can also be deployed to challenge the status quo in unique ways.

As AIDS rates dropped among white gay men, and the advent of anti-retroviral (ARV) therapy transformed what was once a deadly disease into a chronic condition for those living in the Global North, attention shifted to sub-Saharan Africa, which is currently bearing the brunt of the epidemic. At the end of 2013, it was estimated that 70 percent of the approximately 35 million people in the world living with HIV reside in sub-Saharan Africa (Joint United Nations Programme on HIV/AIDS 2014:3). Johannesburg, including Soweto and other surrounding townships, has the distinction of having the highest HIV rate of any city in the world, with an estimated 11 percent of its population (980,000 people) infected (Shisana et al. 2014). As a result, the news media contain numerous images of AIDS orphans, stories of young girls raped by men hoping to be cured of AIDS, and former South African president Thabo Mbeki's denials of HIV as the cause of AIDS. While reports of AIDS in Africa were in part intended to facilitate aid campaigns by highlighting disparity, they have also shaped North American and European views of the continent. AIDS has been "prolifically productive" in reinforcing portrayals of Africans as poor, sick, and ignorant (Comaroff and Comaroff 2011:179). Consequently, AIDS discourse has not transcended but rather mirrored colonial perceptions of Africa.

These renderings are not confined to the popular press but also permeate scientific and public health AIDS narratives. Epidemiological research in sub-Saharan Africa has repeatedly shown that women are most vulnerable to HIV infection (Chersich and Rees 2008). These high rates are blamed in part on men's lack of condom use and women's inability to insist on prophylaxis, particularly if a woman is receiving financial benefits from her sexual partner. As a result, Africans have been perceived as patriarchal, prone to prostitution-like behavior, and unable or unwilling to accept the importance of safe sex (Bibeau and Pederson 2002). Reports that African women insert substances such as snuff into their vaginas to promote "dry sex"—considered to be a risk factor for HIV transmission—exoticize African sexuality. Even as ARVs were hailed as a highly effective treatment for HIV, some doctors asked if they were appropriate for Africa. If Africans were not responsible enough to take ARVs regularly, it was argued, these drugs should not be distributed, as researchers feared an irregular dosing regimen would result in resistant strains of HIV appearing (Harries et al. 2001). These early debates over access to ARVs reinforced previous portrayals of Africans as ignorant, lazy, and undeserving of treatment. And as concerns about the development of treatments and people's access to them continue to constitute a powerful narrative, global health representations of Africans, African behaviors, African risk factors, and African sexuality significantly impact the lives of people throughout the continent.

The effects of these AIDS narratives are particularly tangible in microbicides, which embody biomedical attitudes about African women. Developed to redress what are considered to be endemic African gender disparities, a microbicide gel can in theory be used without the tacit knowledge of a sexual partner (Bell 2003; Mantell, Dworkin, et al. 2006). Much more than an HIV prevention tool, microbicides are medical technologies intended to encourage female autonomy and empowerment. Remarking on this profound potential, Stephen Lewis, UN Special Envoy for HIV/AIDS in Africa, asked attendees at a conference to see microbicides "not merely as one of the great scientific pursuits of the age, but as a significant emancipation for women whose cultural, social and economic inheritance have put them so gravely at risk. Never in human history have so many died for so little reason. You have a chance to alter the course of that history. Can there be any task more noble?" (Lewis 2004). As a result of appeals such as these, microbicides have been increasingly embraced by virologists, AIDS activists, and governmental organizations as pharmaceuticals capable of radically improving the lives of African women. Microbicides are touted not only as solutions to a virus but also a presumed African way of life. Nevertheless, in seeking to liberate women, microbicide advocates constrain their identity through these portrayals and prescribe medical responses to the epidemic.

However, microbicide development is not only motivated by a desire to save the lives of African women; it is also profitable. In a global AIDS industry that is now over three decades old, massive investments have been made in biomedical solutions, propelling research on innovative HIV prevention technologies and attracting sizable donor funding. In 2012, $245 million

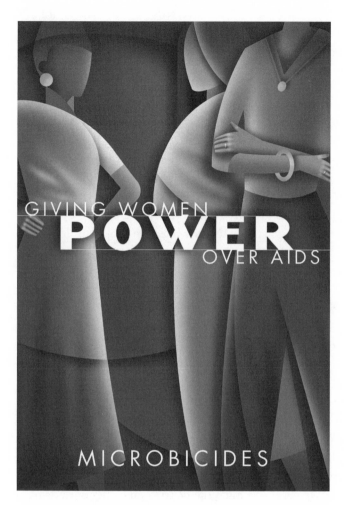

**FIGURE 1.** "Giving women power over AIDS" poster. Courtesy of the International Partnership for Microbicides.

was given toward the research and development of microbicides alone (HIV Vaccines and Microbicides Resource Tracking Working Group 2013). A great deal of this money went to fund clinical trials. A central driver of the pharmaceutical economy, clinical trials are necessary to prove the effectiveness of a new drug and qualify it for licensure by regulatory agencies such as the US Food and Drug Administration (FDA). Often involving thousands of participants, more clinical trials are taking place than ever before. Because of the high cost and numerous guidelines associated with trials in the United States and Western Europe, pharmaceutical companies and research organizations have consistently conducted trials abroad, most notably in the Global South.

As a result, many trials have been portrayed as foreign enterprises, while local communities and participants are cast as relatively powerless, given their low levels of income and education (Craddock 2004; Leger 2008; Löwy 2000; Petryna 2006).

Although the vast majority of microbicide trials have been funded by organizations and agencies in the Global North, they have been carried out in sub-Saharan Africa. Reinforcing characterizations of international trials as neocolonial, African scientists have expressed concerns about foreign "northern experts" who are "not so interested in local needs but in their own research agendas" (Ramsay 2002:1665). Indeed, local scientific contributions toward multisite clinical trials are often restricted to the setting up of sites and the managing of trial populations. Meanwhile, the trial coordinators to whom the data is channeled are located off-site in research institutes and laboratories. Noting that participants are drawn from impoverished populations that lack reliable medical care, critics argue that microbicide trials are made possible through inequality. Meanwhile, clinicians complain that poverty encourages African participants to be dishonest and to cheat by pocketing money for enrollment without taking the drug being tested. In these assessments of the relationship between medical researchers and their subjects, notions of race and morality are embedded into narratives of economy and poverty. Consequently, the significance of clinical trials lies well beyond biomedical results. As clinical trials create close connections between international corporations, pharmaceuticals, governments, and people, responses to innovative biotechnologies constitute an ongoing dialogue about differing social, economic, and political contexts.

Through their very uncertainty, microbicide trials engender optimism. In so doing, trials form a biotechnical embrace, which "creates a popular culture that is enamored with the biology of hope, attracting venture capital that continues even in the face of contemporary constraints to generate new treatment modalities" (DelVecchio Good 2007:377). In 2013, at the Microbicide Trials Network (MTN)'s annual regional meeting in Cape Town, MTN co-chair Sharon Hillier addressed the gathering of site staff, researchers, and scientists, saying that "farmers and microbicide researchers work very hard, and they never, never lose hope." Rather than discouraging research, each successive microbicide trial keeps hope alive, despite the long history of unsuccessful and even harmful trials. Of 37 trials testing 39 HIV prevention strategies, only 5 demonstrated any protection against HIV transmission

(Karim et al. 2010:1168). While microbicide advocates have tirelessly asserted that the technology could radically improve the lives of African women, not a single microbicide formulation has been licensed. After years of testing, only one microbicide gel has proven even marginally effective. Yet investment in microbicides has not dwindled, in part because the pharmaceutical economy is designed to function through the perpetuation of clinical trials rather than the release of a product. Unlike new drugs to treat heart disease, diabetes, or cancer in wealthy nations, a licensed microbicide would be distributed to poor women and not sold at a high profit. Consequently, the hope of finding an effective product is more valuable than actually identifying one.

## HOW TO HAVE THEORY IN A CLINICAL TRIAL

As medical research becomes increasingly viewed as an economically driven enterprise, clinical trials and their organizers are seen as seeking to control vulnerable research participants. Dovetailing with Foucault's (1994) analysis of the development of biomedicine, this interpretation casts medicine as an institution through which bodies are made docile through a strategic deployment of specialized knowledge and procedures. Indeed, the clinical trial enrollment process is designed to prepare participants to adhere to medical instructions while having them consent to regular medical monitoring. Our own research was part of this endeavor. As members of the Social Science Unit of the MDP301's Johannesburg site, we conducted research that was firmly embedded within the trial. Unsurprisingly, the information gathered by the Social Science Unit was to be an additional tool to help trial administrators surveil women's attitudes and bodies. We were charged with collecting information relating to product use and acceptability: Did women like or dislike the gel? Did they experience any problems while using the gel? Were they using the gel as directed? Would they continue to use the gel if the product was proven effective? To answer these questions, we employed a mixed methodology that incorporated quantitative and qualitative approaches to generate detailed information that was also statistically significant (Pool et al. 2010). By the end of the trial, the Johannesburg Social Science Unit had conducted 401 serial in-depth interviews, 44 focus groups, and countless informal interviews in the clinic.[2] But we did not confine our activities to medical settings. Wanting to understand the townships affected by the trials, we engaged in participant observation, hanging out in pool halls, snacking on watermelon at community markets, visiting women's homes, and talking to people at local stores.

Through interviews, focus groups, and many hours spent hanging out in the community, we conclusively documented that participants regarded the gel as highly "acceptable." In only 11 of the 401 in-depth interviews was the gel was deemed "unacceptable."[3] While this simple dichotomy might appeal to some statisticians, we found, as anthropologists often do, that participants' responses were far more complex. Women's narratives were layered with multiple meanings and powerful expressions of female agency. Participants emphasized their personal familiarity with the gel, asserting that they possessed knowledge medical researchers did not. PRO 2000/5, we were often told, worked. Like many participants, Boikanyo reported that the gel cleansed her vagina, prevented infections, and acted as a powerful aphrodisiac. Others claimed that the gel increased fertility, enhanced sexual relationships, and increased love and commitment between intimate partners. Given these positive outcomes, participants often remarked that the gel treated them well and was "good for a great many things." Seeking to improve their general health and well-being, women came to use the gel for reasons other than HIV prevention.

Patients frequently attach signification to pharmaceuticals that transcends the strictly medical (Whyte et al. 2002), but the uncertainty of clinical trials intensifies this process. Using PRO 2000/5, an unproven drug, created a space in which participants had a unique ability to acquire and control knowledge, thereby democratizing medicine. Indeed, MDP301 participants evaluated the gel independently of standardized trial messages, on their own terms. Regardless of the researchers' often strident attempts to regulate the conditions and parameters of pharmaceutical use within a clinical trial, women situated the gel locally, outside of a strictly medical context, in terms of bodily experience, cultural understandings, and social norms. While women invoked a medical discourse about PRO 2000/5's active chemical compounds interacting with human physiology, they also drew from South African beliefs regarding the curative powers of fluids flowing through the body. The physical properties of the gel were an important catalyst of this process. Whereas pills seldom have an immediate effect after ingestion, the gel produced a number of sensations and physiological changes, most notably vaginal lubrication and discharge. Microbicides, particularly those inserted prior to sex, as was the case with PRO 2000/5, are distinctive in their ability to transform bodies.

While the biomedical uncertainty of PRO 2000/5, coupled with the sensations of gel use, encouraged women to make their own meaning, so too did the research process itself. Possessing limited data regarding in vivo use, trial staff relied on the experiences of participants to gather information about the gel. Nurses, doctors, and the members of the Social Science Unit repeatedly told participants that their honesty was critical to the success of the trial. Because women's intimate behaviors could not be physically monitored or observed by the staff, the MDP301 was built around the self-reporting of gel use, vaginal practices, and sexual acts. If participants didn't use the gel, forgot to inform nurses about the results, or lied about their behavior, the trial would fail. Acutely aware of this fact, trial coordinators sought to convey the importance of accurate self-reporting to participants. Through trial interviews such as the ones we were conducting, women quickly came to understand that it was their use of the gel that would ultimately determine the trial's outcome. Elaborating on the statements of trial administrators and noting that they possessed experiential knowledge of the gel that staff did not, participants remarked that rich white researchers were now dependent on poor black women.

Women's narratives were not uncontested. When MDP301 administrators became aware that participants' assertions were far from what microbicide advocates had envisioned, they quickly dismissed these claims as products of rumor and misunderstanding and attempted to "correct" them through radio programs, seminars, and education campaigns. But these actions had little effect. Once the trial ended and PRO 2000/5 was found to be ineffective in preventing HIV, trial researchers were confident that stories of the gel's efficacy would at last cease. They did not. As women continued to resist official explanations, trial coordinators became exasperated. This conflict between the official results and the views of participants is one of many examples of friction that occurred throughout the MDP301. Defining "friction" as the unexpected, unequal, and unstable aspects of global encounters, Tsing (2011) argues that much as a spinning wheel requires friction to move a vehicle forward, asymmetrical and disparate encounters shift established power relationships, propelling them into new territory. Within the context of clinical trials, friction is fostered through the inherent uncertainty of medical testing. Neither doctors nor participants can effectively monopolize knowledge.

Conceptualizing and employing pharmaceuticals in ways unimagined by the product developers, trial participants destabilized many of the inherent suppositions of medical research. Whereas global health often casts African women as an impoverished and vulnerable population that is completely dependent on international interventions for aid and well-being, participants' narratives inverted this relationship. Instead of personifying a population ignorant of *materia medica*, participants presented themselves as knowledgeable and experienced, while portraying trial doctors as lacking substantive knowledge of the pharmaceutical being evaluated. As conventional identities became upended and exchanged, conventional power relationships also shifted. Women like Boikanyo repeatedly asserted that they gained control and felt empowered on the trial. Interestingly, these responses were made possible by the same trial mechanisms that sought to monitor and manage women's bodies: informed consent, randomization, in-depth interviewing, and pharmaceutical usage. Rather than turning women into docile participants, the process of testing an uncertain drug fostered their independence and agency. Consequently, clinical trials are not only controlling but also liberating.

## FERTILE FLOWS

Reframing relationships between participants and trialists as well as between the Global South and the Global North, we ground our analysis in the experiences, perceptions, and beliefs of South African women. Because the participants' claims that the gel was "good for a great many things" resulted in part from the gel's ability to traverse bodily and social boundaries, South African notions of flow serve as a useful metaphor for understanding the productive circulation of knowledge, resources, and experiences between medical researchers, trial participants, and the communities in which they live. Rather than simply acting as a source of misunderstanding or exploitation, international clinical trials create fertile flows in which women are able to find not only empowerment but also salvation. To trace these movements of signification, capital, and encounters, this book is divided into two parts. The first—Chapters 1 and 2—examines the growing relationship between global health and pharmaceutical testing, chronicling the social and scientific production of medical knowledge and how this knowledge propels an interest in, and funding for, new biotechnologies. The remainder of the book—Chapters 3 through 6—explores the ways in which MDP301 participants were able to use the gel and the trial to reimagine their bodies, gender, and sociality.

Examining the processes through which medical narratives construct identity, the first chapter juxtaposes nineteenth-century portrayals of Africans as infested natives with contemporary scientific and global health accounts of HIV/AIDS. In both cases, blackness, disease, sexuality, immorality, and gender are linked in ways that create and perpetuate negative stereotypes of Africans. These assumptions in turn steer the development of new technologies to prevent HIV transmission. Microbicides have been advocated as female-controlled pharmaceuticals that could be used without a man's knowledge, countering women's inability to negotiate condom use. Intended to be much more than an HIV prevention method, microbicides were envisioned as an empowering biotechnology that could positively affect the lives of women throughout Africa. With medical science cast as the solution to African inequality, microbicides medicalize gender disparities while seeking to export Western notions of female empowerment via pharmaceuticals.

Charting the history of randomized clinical trials, the second chapter examines the social, economic, and political contexts of medical testing. To promote standardization and exclude social variables, clinical trials rely on the use of placebos, randomization, double-blinding, and careful statistical analysis. Now considered the gold standard of medical testing, clinical trials have come under repeated scrutiny for their treatment of human subjects. From purposely infecting mentally handicapped children with hepatitis in the 1960s to increasing the risk of HIV infection among southern African women in recent microbicide trials, scientists have been accused of unethically exposing vulnerable and minority populations to life-threatening diseases. In response, medical researchers and pharmaceutical advocates have argued that in times of medical crisis—such as the AIDS pandemic—the need to save lives through rapid drug development and testing outweighs any risk to subjects. Recasting experimental pharmaceuticals as hopeful technologies, the promise of eventual success transforms medical research into everyday good practice. Despite having caused harm to participants, microbicide trials continue to be funded and conducted, as advocates promote their potential to prevent HIV and empower African women.

Chapter 3 follows Mandisa as she joins the MDP301, illustrating the ways in which clinical trials inspire participants to create meaning through their experiences of recruitment, screening, and enrollment. To attract volunteers, trial administrators sought to disseminate standardized messages stressing the value of medical research, the MDP301, and microbicides. However, township residents were dubious and challenged trial narratives.

MDP301 procedures considered routine by medical personnel, such as HIV testing, blood draws, and remuneration, were said to be proof that the trial purposely infected participants with HIV, sold their blood, and employed witchcraft to kill local residents. On one hand, these rumors acted as a powerful counternarrative, warning of the spiritual danger posed by foreign medical researchers. Situating the trial within an environment of postcolonial insecurity, the MDP301 was linked to an occult economy that threatened social reproduction. On the other hand, trial rumors also articulated concerns about the ways in which African women access cash and achieve financial independence. While female participants were believed to be exploited and killed through the MDP301, there was little sympathy for their fate. Demonstrating the unanticipated meanings of pharmaceuticals, the very women whom microbicides were designed to empower were accused of receiving illicit money through the trial without engaging in honest labor. As a result, participants were cast as greedy, dishonest, and immoral.

Shifting attention from the MDP301 as a vehicle for meaning, Chapter 4 examines the way in which women's use of the gel not only shaped experience but also altered gendered relationships. Inserted just prior to sexual intercourse, the gel physically and socially restructured intimate moments between participants and their partners. For many women, the use of vaginal agents was not new. In an effort to increase male enjoyment and, as a result, male devotion, women reportedly employed a variety of products to dry and tighten their vaginas and consented to unlubricated intercourse. Yet while dry sex was an ideal, it was one that few women practiced, as it often resulted in discomfort or pain. Although the gel was a new pharmaceutical, it was quickly integrated into narratives of dry sex. Equated with cleanliness, the gel was viewed as a drying agent despite its lubricating properties. Furthermore, the gel was reputed to act as a powerful aphrodisiac that drove couples to engage in sex more frequently and for longer periods. Men reported that gel sex increased their love and fidelity, while women noted that their newfound ability to orgasm quickly and frequently motivated them to become more confident and assertive, not only with their partners but with men in general.

Focusing on women's responses to the gel, the fifth chapter explores the ways in which competing notions of efficacy are validated and promoted. For medical researchers, effectiveness was to be determined through evidence-based medicine, but trial participants independently evaluated the gel as its users. Based on their bodily reactions, women alleged that PRO 2000/5 not only prevented HIV infection but also cleansed the body, cured infections, and increased fertility. As evidence, participants invoked southern African ontologies of dirt and flow to conclude that the gel visibly removed pollutants and pathogens from their bodies. Women believed that PRO 2000/5 was much more than a potential method to prevent HIV infection, and that it was demonstratively responsible for improving their reproductive and general health. Consequently, the gel was used by some women on a daily basis, independent of their sexual activity. While MDP301 staff attempted to discourage these beliefs and practices, they were unable to do so. Participants actively challenged medical authority, noting that they possessed a far greater experiential knowledge of PRO 2000/5 than did trial researchers. Altering the relationship between researchers and research subjects, women asserted their embodied knowledge and agency in response to the medical uncertainty inherent in pharmaceutical testing.

After enrolling over nine thousand women over two years, the MDP301 ended. Awaiting the results from London, trialists and participants were overwhelmingly hopeful that PRO 2000/5 would prove to be the first effective microbicide. However, this was not to be. The trial was flat, meaning sufficient evidence had been collected to verify that PRO 2000/5 did not affect rates of HIV transmission. Chapter 6 explores the closure of the MDP301 and the release of the results, which inspired a diverse set of responses. Researchers were dispirited but still convinced that microbicides were the solution to Africa's HIV epidemic. The South African media, however, seized on the failure as proof that clinical trials were fundamentally harmful, and that PRO 2000/5 was a toxic pharmaceutical designed to kill Africans. For their part, participants were discouraged by the results but drew a clear distinction between the trial and the product it had tested. PRO 2000/5 might have failed to show efficacy, but for many women the trial was a success. They portrayed themselves as individuals who had risked their healthy bodies through trial participation; in doing so, they had demonstrated their virtue, reconfigured gender relations, and improved their health. Co-opting religious language and experience, these women stated that it was the clinical trial, not the microbicide, which had allowed them to improve their material, social, and spiritual lives.

Medical testing is playing a critical role in shaping contemporary socialities and economies through the proliferation of clinical trials worldwide. Examining developments in microbicide research and global clinical trials, the conclusion charts the evolving trends in medical research. A string of flat trials has fundamentally altered the treatment of participants, with frequent accusations of irregular product usage. Trialists have begun closely monitoring women's bodies for product adherence through intensified blood screenings and applicator testing. As microbicide trialing continues, the dream of empowering African women through pharmaceuticals continues to rely on an economy of hope. Even though it has been proven that antiretroviral microbicides are 39 percent effective in preventing HIV, they have not been marketed, in part because to do so would threaten the funding of ongoing clinical trial research. Profit is gained from testing HIV prevention drugs, not releasing them to an impoverished population.

In combining an analysis of the development, practice, and meaning of biomedical technologies with a detailed ethnography of the lives of South African trial participants and township residents, we seek to shift conceptions of clinical trials from impersonal medical enterprises to intimate exchanges between diverse groups of people. To do this, we employ numerous quotes drawn from informal conversations, interviews, and focus groups, allowing participants to express their thoughts, beliefs, and sentiments in their own words. This reconceptualization is particularly important in clinical settings, which are increasingly denounced as dehumanizing. Perhaps unsurprisingly, the MDP301's substantial social science focus was unprecedented in a clinical trial. A lead investigator in many of South Africa's microbicide trials, Gita Ramjee, commented that the MDP301 remains a unique example of a research model that integrated a social science approach into a larger biomedical enterprise. Not only has this model failed to be replicated in South Africa, it is extremely rare in trials elsewhere. Yet as the following chapters will demonstrate, we believe integrating social science research within the medical realm is, like the gel, good for a great many things.

# Part 1

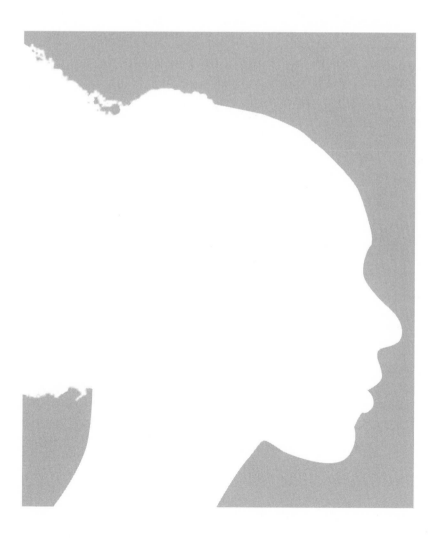

# Infested Natives and Empowering Biotechnologies

An "epidemic of signification" (Treichler 1999), the HIV/AIDS crisis has simultaneously led to the innovation of new diagnostic techniques and biotechnologies while reiterating long-standing narratives of racial difference. Although the initial discovery of AIDS among gay men in the United States led the disease to be associated with homosexuality, by the mid-1980s narratives of "Black Africans" with AIDS began to grab headlines. Now acknowledged as the birthplace of HIV, and home to the highest prevalence rates in the world, sub-Saharan Africa has become a major focus of HIV/AIDS activism, research, and intervention. As cases of HIV in sub-Saharan Africa have continued to rise despite the existence of an effective prevention technology, the condom, the epidemiological profile of AIDS has become increasingly young and female. Almost 70 percent of all HIV-infected women can be found in Africa. These women have a higher chance of HIV infection than men and acquire HIV up to seven years earlier than men (Karim et al. 2012). Statistics such as these have led to the labeling of younger women as a "most at-risk population" (Chersich and Rees 2008). Transcending medical data, many explanations of the continent's high rate of HIV/AIDS focus on a unique "African" sexual culture, in which multiple sexual partners, gender inequalities, and unlubricated sex are common. While these narratives are based on epidemiological models, they nevertheless echo earlier portrayals of degenerate African natives. From European explorers to colonial public health officials, blackness, perverse sexuality, and disease have been inextricably linked.

Casting high rates of HIV as the result of cultural and sexual factors has had important consequences, affecting the development of technology to stem the pandemic. Drawing from the principles and innovations of the birth control movement, AIDS activists have argued for a female-controlled mechanism for prevention. While this is in part a response to epidemiological findings, it is also motivated by assumptions about ingrained gender power imbalances resulting from local cultural beliefs. Vulnerability to infection is attributed to powerlessness, which may include the inability to negotiate for "safer sex" and insist on condom use (Pettifor et al. 2004). In particular, HIV infection is linked to sexual violence (Dunkle et al. 2004a; Maman et al. 2000; Pronyk et al. 2006), which is experienced by 25 percent of South African women (Jewkes et al. 2002). Although condoms are highly reliable barriers against infection, they are impractical for women to use under such circumstances (Wilkinson 2002a). Christopher J. Elias and Lori Heise (1993:1; emphasis added), two microbicide advocates, declare, "Underlying gender power inequities severely limit the ability of many women to protect themselves from HIV infection, especially in the absence of a prevention technology they can use, when necessary, *without their partner's consent.*" Consequently, new technologies have been sought that women can use without the knowledge or approval of men.

While initially championed only by reproductive health advocates, microbicides have come to be seen as the ideal female-controlled prevention method. Unlike condoms, which require male cooperation, microbicides "put the power to protect in women's hands" because they can be used clandestinely, or without the explicit acquiescence of a partner (GCM 2016). Thought to support autonomy in sexual decision-making and, therefore, in HIV prevention, microbicides are touted as products capable of realigning gendered inequalities and women's vulnerability to HIV infection (Bell 2000; Mantell, Dworkin, et al. 2006). Microbicides have thus been labeled the "gel of hope" in the press. But while microbicides are a new biotechnology, they also embody and address enduring beliefs that Africans are fundamentally at risk and in need. These assumptions create hierarchical relationships, relegating African women to the role of victims at the margins of what appears to be vital medical research.

## MEDICAL REVOLUTIONS REEXAMINED

The protocols, tools, and assumptions of medical practice have been constructed through lengthy and complex processes. Often focusing on "great men" such as Andreas Vesalius, William Harvey, or Robert Koch, many histories of medicine depict the discipline as the ceaseless accumulation of physiological and biological knowledge, advancing along a single trajectory. However, this orderly portrayal overlooks many of the circuitous and contradictory paths that medicine has taken. Rather than viewing medicine as simply a string of innovations by great (white) men, we must look at the ways in which European concerns regarding morality, conquest, and race have guided it. Medicine embodies social norms and aspirations that continue to assert themselves in contemporary health crises. Two eras of "revolution" are particularly important for contextualizing responses to the HIV/AIDS epidemic: (1) the use of scientific explanations to make sense of racial difference and (2) the advent of germ theory and the subsequent rise of public health. While the imperial ambitions of European nations played a critical role in each of these eras, this influence is largely absent in many popular retellings.

Prior to the scientific revolution, health was thought to be maintained through a balance of substances or humors in the body. Popular throughout ancient Greece, Rome, and the Islamic world, humoral theories formed the bedrock of medical practice (Arikha 2007). Illness was attributed to a wide range of causes, including an imbalance of humors or a noxious "bad air" or miasma. Cholera epidemics were regularly attributed to miasmas, as was the Black Death. By the Middle Ages, these beliefs were firmly linked to Christianity, which had long associated sin with disease, and illness with God's judgment and will. Each of the Seven Deadly Sins corresponded to a medical condition, and illness was often viewed as a direct reflection of individual morality (Thomas 1997:16). In the sixteenth and seventeenth centuries, outbreaks of the bubonic plague were simultaneously attributed to evil humors and retribution for sin (Reiser 1985:7; Thomas 1997:18). Notions of miasma and sin would undergird European health beliefs for centuries, and their specters continue to linger in contemporary medical discourse. But these ideas did not exist in isolation. They were given meaning, in part, through their ability to make sense of what would come to be known as racial difference.

Beginning with the search for direct trade routes to Asia by the Portuguese at the end of the fifteenth century, western European nations increasingly came into contact with foreign places and peoples. With the "discovery" of the Americas and the Spice Islands, economic voyages spawned tales of exotic lands, while specimens of newfound flora and fauna sparked a growing interest in ontologies. By the close of the seventeenth century, when Enlightenment ideals had a firm hold on European thought, Europeans were favoring reason (in approaches such as a fledgling scientific method) over the assumptions of the past as they tried to understand the world they were traversing. Seeking to impose a regularity and logic onto the natural world, scholars sorted plants and animals into genera and species. In *Systema Naturae* (1735), Carl Linnaeus, like others of his time, extended the interest in speciation to humanity, which he divided into five taxa: *Americanus*, *Asiaticus*, *Africanus*, *Europeanus*, and *Mostrosus*. While Linnaeus claimed that this classification was scientifically based on phenotypic features, it was also grounded in popular European notions. Drawing from medical beliefs, it associated each race with a different humor: sanguine, choleric, phlegmatic, and melancholic. While *Europeanus* was described as active and adventurous, *Africanus* was cast as lazy and crafty (Graves 2001:39).

Instead of Enlightenment ideals universally dispelling the myths of the past, newfound scientific language perpetuated assumptions about human difference. Biology was one tool through which not only physical variation but also social difference was explained, and racial characteristics were repeatedly linked to intelligence, morality, and social behavior. While skin color was a dominant phenotype in these classifications, cranial and sexual characteristics were widely invoked as indicators of the savageness of particular populations. A high cranial capacity was equated with intelligence, leading to research documenting the acumen of Europeans in contrast to the stupidity of Africans. Drawing from claims that Africans possessed the lowest cranial volume of any race, Georges Cuvier argued that the "Negro" should be viewed as between Europeans and the "most ferocious apes" (quoted in Comaroff 1993:309). For some Europeans, these differences were so extreme that they equated race with species. Scientific racism promoted a hierarchy that justified European social, economic, and political domination of other peoples. Affirming the biological, intellectual, and moral preeminence of Europeans transformed colonialism, segregation, and slavery into excusable institutions.

Genitals and sexual responsiveness were also employed as further evidence of fundamental biological differences between races. The interest in sexual behavior was presented as scientific necessity rather than prurience. In North America, indigenous men allegedly lacked facial hair and possessed small penises, and their sexual drive was thought to be well below that of European men. Explorers and colonists also popularized reports of men wearing the clothes of women and marrying other men. Casting Native American men as feminine and impotent, these tales were cited as proof of the moral and social depravity of an entire race that, it was assumed, would be eventually subjugated by the more masculine and dominant European colonizers (Lyons and Lyons 2004:26). In contrast to Native Americans, Africans were the embodiment of excessive sexuality, and credited with having large penises as early as the fifteenth century. Measuring African genitalia became a scientific pursuit (Lyons and Lyons 2004:28). Like cranial capacity, penis size was regarded as proof that Africans were evolutionarily closer to the great apes than other humans. Female reproductive anatomy was also cited. Charles White (1799:58–61) stated that African women menstruated more than apes and baboons but less than European women, demonstrating a "regular gradation" among the species. The supposed similarity between apes and Africans led some to assert that sexual relationships between these groups were to be expected. Thomas Jefferson, for example, mentioned stories of apes having intercourse with negresses (Lyons and Lyons 2004:40). From the eighteenth century through the Victorian era, animal and African sexuality were linked, and Africans were associated with wild, exotic, irrational, and immoral sexual practices (Gausset 2001:510; Gilman 1985).

These sexual aberrations were seen as symptomatic of not only the social but also physical afflictions believed to be plaguing an entire continent and its people. In contrast to many temperate regions (such as North America) where introduced diseases had decimated local populations, the seeming ubiquity of deadly infectious diseases in tropical Africa (such as malaria and sleeping sickness) led the continent to be labeled White Man's Grave. Attributing these diseases to miasma, many Europeans viewed foreign environments and the people who inhabited them as pathological. The presence of disease was also blamed in part on African bodies, which were thought to radiate polluting and noxious organisms—natives were characterized as "infested," "greasy," and "indistinguishable from the pestilential surroundings" (Comaroff 1993:316). Merging notions of miasma and sinful illness with scientific racism allowed Europeans to portray Africa and her people as fundamentally diseased. While illness continued to be interpreted in part as punishment for immoral acts such as aberrant sexuality, it also became linked to environment and biology, which in turn was inextricably associated with racial identity.

Beliefs in miasma and scientific racism would gradually be dispelled as another wave of scientific "revolution" rolled through Europe at the end of the nineteenth century. Building on the development of laboratory science, the work of Louis Pasteur and Robert Koch ushered in germ theory. With the discovery of microorganisms, disease was reframed as the work of bacteria or other pathogens. The advent of germ theory reshaped not only how illness was viewed but also its treatment and prevention. Unlike an intangible ill wind, a discrete infectious agent could potentially be restricted or contained, thereby limiting future infections. This change paved the way for the development of public health, "the science and art of preventing disease, prolonging life and promoting physical health and efficiency through organized community efforts for the sanitation of the environment, the control of community infections, the education of the individual in principles of personal hygiene . . ." (Winslow 1920:30). But despite the paradigm shift from miasma to germs and an endorsement of the science of disease prevention, popular notions of illness and morality continued to permeate medical discourse. In the United States, tuberculosis campaigns mirrored evangelical exhortations to repent and to embrace salvation (Tomes 1999). Educational pamphlets were referred to as "catechisms" and contained "commandments" that equated hygienic practices with God's natural law (Tomes 1997:279).

As public health approaches were exported to Europe's and America's foreign possessions, the creation and implementation of medical programs were profoundly impacted by the changing colonial context. By the nineteenth century, European governments had transformed the small settlements initially established as refueling stations and trading outposts into full-fledged colonies. To sustain colonial rule over vast areas of land inhabited by diverse peoples, a permanent and stable European presence was required. As governments relied on settlers to control their colonial possessions, the need to decrease white mortality rates prompted the first earnest scientific study of diseases associated with equatorial regions. Consequently, a new field of tropical medicine was developed and embraced in an ongoing partnership between medical professionals and colonial officials. The London School of Tropical Medicine was considered a "de facto medical department of the colonial office" (Worboys 1990:25). This association with European political and economic domination has led to the labeling of tropical medicine as a "fundamentally imperialistic" discipline (Farley 1991:3). As medical researchers identified the pathogens responsible for past epidemics, health officials introduced a range of sanitation and residential guidelines aimed at arresting the future spread of disease. These in turn provided colonial officials a new tool to govern through the medical control of bodies. Invoking germ theory and employing health protocols such as quarantine allowed governments not only to preserve the health of Europeans but also to segregate non-Europeans. Medical discourse was used not only to reinforce conceptual boundaries between whites and blacks, but also to create physical ones.

These new health discourses and interventions were aided by the burgeoning notion of culture. In an attempt to finally bring an end to scientific racism, Franz Boas (1904; 1911) argued that human variation should be understood not in terms of biology but rather culture. Unlike French ideas of *civilisation*, which cast humankind as a single whole striving to attain greater levels of progress and betterment, the German *kultur* stressed not the similarities but rather the variations between people (Kuper 1999). Acquired through socialization rather than genetics, culture provided a way of conceptualizing difference without invoking biology. But as narratives of racial difference shifted from biology to culture, several assumptions remained in place. Like explanations advocating the biological determination of race, popular notions of culture cast groups as subject to factors that are largely beyond individual control, such as social conditioning. In some ways, culture was a more effective tool for making sense of difference than race because it could draw on a Lamarckian paradigm—in which organisms could consciously adapt and then transmit these acquired characteristics to their offspring—which had been discredited in the natural sciences (Malik 1996:159). Accounting for human differences in a way that biological theories of the time could not, culture was transformed into "a functionally equivalent substitute for the older idea of 'race temperament'" (Stocking 1982:265). Although the original intent had been to refute scientific racism, "we have a 'new racism' in which 'culture,' 'tradition' and 'ethnicity' perform the work previously achieved by the category of 'race'" (Macleod and Durrheim 2002:788).

Whereas Africans had been regarded as less developed humans that could potentially "catch up" to Europeans, cultural explanations recast Africans as intrinsically different, particularly in regards to health behaviors (Jochelson 2001:123). This shift was embraced by public health officials, who used medical interventions coupled with cultural explanations as tools of segregation. As South Africa's first national health measure—one that would remain in effect until 1977—the Public Health Act (1919) advocated racial separation as a primary means of preventing communicable disease (Phillips 1990). White concerns that a large metropolitan black population would lead to poor sanitation and increased illness rates led to the establishment of stricter influx controls (Comaroff and Comaroff 1992:229). After the Second World War, rising rates of venereal disease prompted measures that heavily incorporated cultural explanations. It was argued that Africans living in cities were at much greater risk for contracting and spreading syphilis because the native population was "culturally unsuited" to urban living (Jochelson 2001). Once Africans migrated to urban centers, the cultural norms believed to control the natural sexual impulses of Africans were thought to be lost, leading to increased rates of promiscuity and higher incidences of syphilis. Once again, black migration to urban areas was restricted to preserve public health. In South Africa and elsewhere, medicine became one of the primary ways through which the relationships between white and nonwhite bodies were managed. As with earlier discussions regarding cranial capacity and sexuality, public health guidelines were rationalized through a seemingly scientific discourse. Today, these narratives and resulting power relationships have been modified and adapted to produce responses to the HIV/AIDS pandemic.

## AN AFRICAN VIRUS

The historical propensity to hypersexualize black bodies, cast them as fundamentally diseased, and attribute high morbidity to the inflexibility of African culture deeply underpins medical and public health responses to the AIDS crisis. While teams of scientists were frantically seeking to discover a disease agent for what would come to be known as AIDS, researchers worked to understand the origins and the natural history of the disease. Initially, it seemed that AIDS afflicted only gay men in the United States, but as the epidemic worsened, other risk groups were identified. Famously known as the four Hs, homosexuals, hemophiliacs, heroin users, and Haitians were the initial subjects of AIDS research (Treichler 1999). These populations were linked through a grand epidemiological narrative in which AIDS had spread from Haiti to the United States (or the other way around) via sex tourism, and then gay men who had donated blood or taken drugs intravenously transmitted the disease to those groups.

But this model began to be challenged in 1983, when the first cases of "Black Africans" with AIDS were popularized, which then led to a number of earlier deaths being retrospectively diagnosed (Preda 2004:88). Three years later, a paper published in the *Lancet* claimed that there was evidence that HIV had been present in African populations as early as 1959 (Nahmias et al. 1986). These cases quickly led to the adoption of "Africans" as a risk group. In comparison to the four Hs, "Africans" was a much broader category. By the 1990s, the rate of HIV in sub-Saharan Africa had increased dramatically. While the incidence of infection in countries could vary significantly—between less than 1 percent in some countries to over 15 percent in others—"Africa" became synonymous with the AIDS pandemic. As a result, AIDS seemed to transcend the label of sexually transmitted infection and adopt the characteristics of a tropical and African illness. Resembling its role in earlier colonial portrayals, the entire continent south of the Sahara continued to be cast "as a (potentially unlimited) reservoir of disease," with a range of severe viruses such as Ebola, Marburg, and yellow fever described as "African" (Preda 2004:86). Given the evidence, AIDS appeared to be another chapter in the long saga of deadly African diseases. This narrative was embraced by medical researchers and the media alike. The opening scene in the HBO movie *And the Band Played On*, which retells the early years of the AIDS epidemic, begins with the protagonist witnessing the effects of an Ebola outbreak in Zaire.

As doctors and researchers sought explanatory and epidemiological models to make sense of the Africa epidemic, ingrained assumptions regarding blackness, tropical disease, sexuality, and culture came to the fore. In postulating the origin of HIV in the 1980s, explanations of the mechanism through which the virus "jumped" from animals to humans tended to focus on sexual and cultural practices. Theories included sexual practices involving the use of monkey blood (Karpas 1987) and the possibility that Africans had had intercourse with monkeys (Sabatier 1988:50). Although initially there was little scientific data to support these claims, they were disseminated in both scientific and popular publications. Seeking explanations for high rates of HIV, researchers pointed to a number of "African" practices, including a widow having intercourse to remove her dead husband's spirit (Campbell and Kelly 1995; Chipfakacha 1997), levirate and sororate marriages (Sow et al. 1998), polygamy (Cleland and Ferry 1995), and witchcraft (Yamba 1997; Boahene 1996) or traditional healing (Peltzer et al. 2006), as well as attitudes such as an indifference to chastity. The belief that Africans did not value virginity or monogamy was popularized in part by the work of John C. Caldwell, Pat Caldwell, and Pat Quiggin (1989:195), who wrote, "The evidence is that Africans neither placed aspects of sexual behavior at the center of their moral and social systems nor sanctified chastity." The assumption that Africans have a tendency to engage in higher rates of multipartner sex can still be found throughout HIV/AIDS research (Stillwaggon 2003).

While many of these early assertions have been subsequently discredited, an interest in exotic African sexuality continues to permeate HIV narratives through discussions of transactional sex, dry sex, and circumcision. Citing ethnographies such as that of E. E. Evans-Pritchard (1974:113), Caldwell et al. (1989:203) note that "transactions relating to sexual activity have been looked upon in Africa as equally normal as those relating to work, and it is their absence rather than their presence that is likely to arouse surprise or even disgust." Beginning the 1990s, accounts of women engaging in "transactional sex" have been documented more extensively by researchers and it is now considered one of the leading risk behaviors for contracting HIV (Dunkle et al. 2004b). Parallel with these stories, researchers began documenting what came to be known as "dry sex"—unlubricated intercourse. Africans were portrayed as having a strong preference for dry sex, a practice thought to cause the vagina to tear, thereby making women more susceptible to HIV infection (Brown et al. 1993; Runganga and Kasule 1995). Although researchers are no longer measuring penises, there continues to be a great deal of interest in African sexuality, including male genitalia. Recently, a number of studies were conducted to determine if circumcision would reduce the risk of HIV infection (Weiss et al. 2008), although the low "cultural acceptability" of the procedure is regarded as a barrier to broad implementation (Westercamp and Bailey 2007). Detractors argue that male circumcision results in unrestrained and rampant sexuality on the part of those who are circumcised, undoing the gains made in transforming gender in southern African societies (Kalichman et al. 2007).

Reading these documents, one can easily get the impression that Africans have unique sexual practices, especially compared with those of Europeans and North Americans. Furthermore, African culture is explicitly regarded as a key influence on the sexual choices of individuals. Leclerc-Madlala (2001a:41) writes that "Zulu sexual culture" is characterized by "gender inequity, transactional sex, the socio-cultural *isoka* ideal of multiple sexual partnerships, lack of discussion on matters of sexuality in the home and between sexual partners, the conditioning of both men and women to accept sexual violence as 'normal' masculine behavior along with the 'right' of men to control sexual encounters, and the existence of increasingly discordant and contested gender scripts." The United Nations Economic Commission for Africa published a report stating that culture plays a "major role" in the following behaviors: gender inequalities, wife inheritance and widow cleansing, polygamy, domestic violence, and "harmful practices like female genital mutilation" (UNECA 2008:18–20). The report, like others, portrays African culture as either contributing to or functioning as the primary cause of high rates of HIV/AIDS on the continent (Bibeau and Pedersen 2002; Briggs 2005; Treichler 1991).

These narratives of culture tend to emphasize four main features. The first is that of a single "African" culture that is applied as if the region were an undifferentiated whole (Stillwaggon 2003:812). In the context of HIV/AIDS research, statements such as this are common: "Despite the differences between Africans from different cultures in terms of geography, linguistics, religiosity and ways of life, there is a dominant socio-religious philosophy shared by all Africans" (van Dyk 2001:61). Secondly, medical researchers tend to view culture as both static and homogenous (Kleinman and Benson 2006:835). A third important tendency is to cast culture as an almost inflexible force that is difficult if not impossible to alter. When analyzing "communities of color," culture is often seen as "a fixed monolithic essence that directs the actions of community members" (Volpp 2000:94). Finally, culture is believed to act as a barrier to substantial behavior change. Consequently, from a biomedical perspective, culture is generally viewed as limiting, rather than empowering, health outcomes (Fox and Swazey 1984; Gordon 1988; Taylor 2007). In linking "African" culture and illness—and as a result race and illness—these narratives mimic those of the nineteenth century, in which black bodies were routinely equated with "degradation, disease, and contagion" (Comaroff 1993:306). Furthermore, behavioral explanations focusing on culture as a leading contributor to high rates of HIV seem to provide scientific and medical proof that African culture is not only different but also pathological. As Briggs (2005:276) writes, "Using liberal languages of multiculturalism, cultural features are pathologized by linking them to notions of biomedical causation." Highlighting "troubling" behaviors, notably sexual practices, and then attributing these proclivities to culture conflates morality, race, and illness.

Focusing on explanations that stress the role of culture and sexuality in this manner has important consequences for HIV/AIDS research and intervention efforts. While concern with sexual practices does appear justified in a pandemic where most cases of HIV transmission occur through sexual contact and sexual actions, Stillwaggon (2003:818) notes, "By framing AIDS in Africa as something that results from an exotic and exceptional sexuality, it has restricted the scope of acceptable research to sexual behavior (and social phenomena that influence partner change, such as migration and gender relations) and circumscribed the actions taken to address the epidemic (problem solving)." The emphasis on sexual encounters has created a tendency to focus on gender relationships and intimate partner interactions. Although health researchers are moving away from views that focus exclusively on culture, these perspectives continue to exert a significant legacy in HIV research, initiatives, and funding through gendered and rights-based discourses. A critical example can be found in narratives regarding condom use as a prevention technique.

In 1987, almost one hundred years after the invention of the rubber condom, the US surgeon general recommended the use of condoms to prevent HIV, particularly for people who were unaware of each other's sexual histories (Youssef 1993). These recommendations were based on solid evidence: condoms are highly efficacious as a barrier at the level of a virus, and consistent use of condoms results in an 80 percent reduction in HIV incidence (Wilkinson 2002a). Condoms were thus viewed as a primary tool through which HIV infection could be prevented in sub-Saharan Africa. In 1995, South Africa's first National AIDS Plan called for condom use as the best available method to fight the epidemic (Bermudes Ribiero Da Cruz 2004:136). As HIV prevalence grew, the number of condoms distributed to sub-Saharan Africa increased from 18 million in 1990 to 236 million in 1998 and approximately 450 million in 2006 (Iliffe 2006:70). Yet despite an ever-growing number of condoms being made available, the rates of HIV infection seem to be unaffected. Although the condom is heralded as the flagship of HIV prevention, it is widely recognized that condoms have limited effectiveness at the population level in terms of the spread of HIV. In explaining the failure of condoms to stem the pandemic, researchers echo Leclerc-Madlala's statement regarding Zulu sexual culture (Dunkle et al. 2004a; Jewkes et al. 2003; Wood et al. 1998). In their narratives, unevenness in condom use results from power dynamics within relationships that undermine women's choices, thereby placing women at risk of HIV infection (Thege 2009). Although statements postulating intercourse between Africans and apes are a thing of the past, contemporary views of HIV risk and prevention technologies are still imbued with the assumption that African sexuality is structured by unique cultural beliefs and is thus nonnormative.

## FEMALE-CONTROLLED MECHANISMS

As narratives regarding the reluctance of men to use condoms and the vulnerability of women to HIV became widespread, advocacy groups began focusing more of their studies on women. At the International Conference on Population and Development held in Cairo in 1994, global leaders committed to championing technologies that would bolster women's right to protection from HIV. In the post-Cairo era, advocates and researchers formed alliances to search for these technologies (Bell 2000). Yet, the idea that biomedical technologies could transform gender relations originated much earlier, in the birth control movement of the 1900s, which heralded contraceptives as a means of female empowerment (Bell 2000; Kaler 2004). As colonial notions of race and illness pervaded contemporary notions regarding HIV, so too did feminist assumptions regarding female-controlled prevention mechanisms. By the early 1980s, two new "female-controlled mechanisms" were being discussed: the female condom and microbicides. While the former would demonstrate its ability to prevent HIV infection, it would be deemed unpopular and would be largely abandoned. In contrast, the hope of microbicides continues to captivate researchers and funders despite the fact that this technology has yet to be conclusively proven effective.

Given the uneven success of male condoms, new barrier methods were explored that aimed to shift decision-making from men to women. One of these was the female condom. Launched in 1984, it was regarded as "a new technology which offered the promise, however distant, of enabling women to take care of themselves in sexual terms, and thus to empower themselves in this context" (Kaler 2004:142). Fashioned from polyurethane—a lighter, more sensitive, and more robust material than latex—the female condom resembled an oversized male condom, open at one end and closed at the other, with a ring to fit in the cervix. In 1991, the FDA approved the female condom for distribution and by 2009 the Joint United Nations Programme on HIV/AIDS (UNAIDS), World Health Organization (WHO), and United Nations Population Fund (UNFPA) had endorsed it, noting that "the female condom in particular is currently the only technology that gives women greater control over protecting themselves from HIV, other STIs and unintended pregnancy" (Peters et al. 2010). In contrast, other barrier methods, such as the diaphragm or cervical cap, have enjoyed significantly less success as HIV protection methods. A multisite trial that assessed the efficacy of the diaphragm in preventing HIV infection found no additional protective effect with use (Padian et al. 2007).[1]

Notwithstanding these endorsements, as well as numerous studies reporting its acceptability among women users, the female condom did not achieve much popularity and support (Hardon 2012; Kaler 2004). In the United States this was partly attributable to the response in the popular media that parodied the device, comparing it to a "jellyfish, a windsock, a fire hose, a colostomy bag, a Baggie, gumboots, a concertina, a plastic freezer bag, something to line Boston's Inner Harbor with, a cross between a test tube and a rubber glove, Edvard Munch's *The Scream*, something designed for a female elephant, something out of the science-fiction cartoon *The Jetsons*, a raincoat for a Slinky toy, or a 'contraption used to punish fallen virgins in the Dark Ages'" (Kaler 2004:144). Some detractors even argued that American women "don't want to be empowered in the bedroom. In the boardroom, yes, but in the bedroom they don't want to jeopardize not having sex with that man" (Herman 1998). The lackluster reaction to the device was reflected in its level of funding: according to an analysis of European and US donor spending on HIV prevention, investments in male and female condom programs dropped significantly between 2000 and 2008, but increased massively for vaccine and microbicide research (Hardon 2012; Peters et al. 2010).

In southern Africa, where there was a far greater sense of urgency for devices women could use and control, the female condom was regarded as a viable and acceptable alternative to the male condom. Several studies established its practicability, in particular for sex workers, who saw the advantages of using hidden devices while charging clients the higher rates for unprotected sex (Wojcicki and Malala 2001). It has been claimed in anecdotes that the clients of sex workers are often too drunk to detect the presence of the female condom.[2] Although the female condom cost significantly more than the male condom, this was offset to a certain extent by its potential for reuse. A study among sex workers in South Africa reported that 83 percent of those interviewed would reuse the female condom (Pettifor et al. 2001). The female condom was even remodeled as an anti-rape device. The Rape-aXe is a female condom embedded with sharp barbs on the inside to snag the rapist's penis. The inventor, Sonnet Ehlers, having encountered many rape victims in her work for a South African blood bank, wanted to send a warning to potential assailants (*Daily Mail* 2010). Despite public enthusiasm for the device, it has not been widely distributed in the public health sector.[3] This mirrors responses to the female condom in general. Although it is effective, can be made more cost effective, and is regarded as acceptable by many, the female condom is not celebrated as a method for women in South Africa.

Around the same time as the development and marketing of the female condom, in the early to mid-1980s, the idea of a microbicide to prevent HIV acquisition first surfaced (Malow et al. 2000; Mantell et al. 2005; Minnis and Padian 2005; Stein et al. 2003). While scientific advances in identifying and mapping the virus that causes AIDS made microbicides as a prevention technology possible, the movement was also driven by an ideology of social medicine and female empowerment. Zena Stein, a key figure in the early advocacy of microbicide technology, believed that biomedical interventions could have profound social effects. Having grown up in South Africa, Stein entered medicine after the Second World War with the conviction that this would enable her and her epidemiologist husband, Mervyn Susser, to make an impact "on the inequalities and injustices of the society we knew" (Wilcox 2003:498). Reflecting on her experiences, Stein said:

> The scene in which we grew up was two separate societies—poor blacks, and middle-class and wealthy whites. So, it was a good situation to learn and think, if you had a social conscience of any kind.
>
> And then there was World War II. By the end of the war, I knew I had to work in some context that would make a difference to society. I took up medicine with the idea that medicine was the way to do something for the poorer populations. (Quoted in Wilcox 2003:498)

The couple followed closely in the footsteps of public health specialists Sidney and Emily Kark, known for piloting the first community-oriented primary care systems in rural KwaZulu-Natal in the 1940s (Tollman 1991). Of Sidney Kark, Stein remarked, "He was the one who explained to us how work as a doctor could in fact do something to society" (Wilcox 2003:499).

Stein worked predominantly on nutrition up until the 1980s, when the first cases of AIDS were reported in New York. While at Columbia University's Mailman School of Public Health, Stein witnessed the devastation caused by the epidemic to the gay community there. Unlike many others at the time, Stein foresaw the possibility of AIDS becoming a crisis among women through heterosexual intercourse. In an interview, Stein talked about the struggle to raise awareness of the threat that AIDS posed to women at a time when the epidemic was regarded as solely a gay problem. Illustrating the potential for cross-infection, she observed that men who had sex with men also had sex with women. Later, she noted that "people didn't really believe us. It took time and effort and continually saying 'Well, women do get it this way.'" My proposal to the NIH [National Institutes of Health] for further study was turned down because 'it [AIDS] wasn't a woman's disease'" (Curry 2003). The publication of Stein's article "HIV Prevention: The Need for Methods Women Can Use" in the *American Journal of Public Health* is regarded as a milestone in the evolution of ideas about HIV prevention. Stein was convinced that hegemonic male sexuality could be challenged by the introduction of a female-controlled prophylaxis, such as a microbicide: "The proposition of this paper is that the empowerment *of* women is crucial for the prevention of HIV transmission *to* women. It follows that prophylaxis must include procedures that rely on the woman and are under her control. A wider range of chemical and physical barriers that block transmission through the vaginal route must be developed and tested" (1990:460). Stein's project sought to link science and activism to impact the lives of women positively. However, this approach was met with considerable resistance. According to anthropologist Ida Susser (2002), Stein's daughter, the draft of her mother's article was initially rejected by several journals and eventually published despite opposition from reviewers.

While activist support for microbicides to protect women against HIV was growing by the early 1990s, as was interest among scientists working on reproductive health, the idea was not popular outside of those circles, especially in the United States. The people with AIDS in America were predominantly male and gay, and the emergent African epidemic had not reached the attention of US researchers and policy makers—or, if indeed it had, it was not regarded as an important issue for national security. This bias toward solving the domestic AIDS epidemic shaped NIH funding, directing research toward prevention among gay men (Karim et al. 2012:489). It was only in 1996, at the Vancouver International AIDS Conference, that the first public announcement of US funding for microbicide research was made. However, at this time, funds were scarce and there was little conviction that a topical microbicide would be feasible or even scientifically viable (Harrison 2011). Microbicide advocates argued that the initial difficulty in finding investments was due to "social and political challenges" that had confronted earlier developments of reproductive health technologies, given the controversy "surrounding matters of sexuality, reproduction and women's empowerment," as well as the "historic bias against scientific endeavors addressing women's health" (Boonstra 2000). Bias against microbicides was equated with bias against women and women's issues.

As a result of the association between microbicides and women's empowerment, the first sustained interest in the technology came primarily from reproductive health specialists, not scientists. The globally networked US-based Population Council was the site of the formation of the Women's Health Advocates on Microbicides (WHAM) in the early 1990s (Bell 2003). Although acknowledgment of the feminization of the AIDS epidemic was growing, the public health research agenda favored vaccines rather than another prevention technology that could be misused or disregarded, as was the case with condoms. Reflecting on the early years of the microbicide movement, Lori Heise (2016), an advocate, researcher, and founder of the Global Campaign for Microbicides, notes, "The irony was that the very community of folks who you would have thought would have joined the effort—those working in HIV—were the least receptive to the message that current strategies were inadequate, especially for women. At the time our allies were women's health advocates and those working on women's sexual and reproductive health; early research was undertaken by those developing contraceptives, not virologists or visionaries in the HIV community." Consequently, the initial discoveries were from the field of contraception rather than virology or immunology (Bell 2003).

As individuals and institutions from the contraceptive industry became involved with microbicides, early formulations were drawn from existing contraceptive technologies, making the continuities between the development of female-controlled contraception and microbicides not only ideological but also scientific. Initial microbicide compounds used the same chemicals as those found in spermicides, such as nonoxynol-9, which had already been used in conjunction with the cervical cap and was added to male condom lubricants. The products in the first generation were chosen because they were already available as spermicides, were reasonably priced, and had shown in vitro activity against HIV (Van Damme 2004). Despite these efforts, the prospect of finding an effective product continued to be slim.

The scientific community regarded microbicides as problematic to test because of their complexity and caricatured them as "a bunch of jams and jellies" (Heise 2009). Criticism also came, somewhat surprisingly, from women's health advocates. The support of reproductive rights advocates had helped build momentum for microbicides, but the Population Council's involvement in the early development of the field caused opponents to fear the employment of microbicides for population control. Feminists also wanted to avoid shifting responsibility for the epidemic to women—a potential result of creating a technological intervention solely for women. Public health officials viewed microbicides as an unreliable technology that could challenge and supplant condoms, and harbored misgivings about microbicide availability, including the possibility of so-called condom migration—a reduction in condom use—even though condoms are more efficacious than microbicides.[4] Similarly, some argued that microbicides would result in risk disinhibition, meaning that women could mislead themselves into thinking that they were protected and subsequently potentially contract HIV at even greater rates. These concerns were routinely dismissed by microbicide activists.

## PROMOTING THE TECHNOLOGY OF EMPOWERMENT IN THE GLOBAL SOUTH

In its initial stages, the field of female-controlled technologies was part of a broader women's health movement, but by the mid-1990s, a new alignment between the international women's coalition and family planning groups, coupled with a shift in discourses of women's health to a human rights framework, led reproductive scientists and advocates to cooperate in discussions on how to accelerate the development of microbicides (Bell 2003). This was accomplished by linking microbicides to the goal of female empowerment. As Quarraisha Abdool Karim, Hilton Humphries, and Zena Stein remark, the search for a microbicide was a movement for women and, initially, to a large extent by women; the technology emerged organically in the context of gatherings and "numerous discussions convened by scientists, feminists, artists and political groups in the USA and from developing countries" (Karim et al. 2012:489). Microbicide meetings were notable for the inclusion of community representatives, advocates, and occasionally former trial participants (McGregor et al. 2013). Casting microbicides as "empowering technologies" in the war against HIV resulted in a rapid increase in the advocacy, research, and development of microbicides (Bell 2003; Bell 2000; Kutikuppala et al. 2004; Mantell, Dworkin, et al. 2006; Mantell et al. 2005). This approach succeeded in combining the outlook of the women's movement with notions regarding the power of culture in non-Western settings.

By the late 1990s, organizations advocating for the development and testing of microbicides were on the rise. Officially launched at the Geneva International AIDS Conference, the Global Campaign for Microbicides (GCM) was established in 1998 and until 2012 was central to galvanizing interest in microbicides. Based in Washington, Nairobi, and Johannesburg, the GCM promoted the development of ideas, political buy-in, and civil society engagement. Also in 1998, the Alliance for Microbicide Development was set up by medical anthropologist Polly Harrison to create relationships between pharmaceutical companies, scientists, advocacy groups, and donors, while bolstering funding opportunities (Harrison 1999). Soon a number of microbicide conferences were also launched. Begun in Berlin in 2000 and held biennially until 2012, the International Microbicides Conference was broadly inclusive, with behavioral and social science tracks, as well as a "community" track, a subset of the basic science and clinical medicine tracks. A primary narrative in the microbicide movement is the involvement of both scientists and women's health activists from the beginning of the development process. Groups such as WHAM note that they provide a forum for scientists and activists to discuss the means of designing female-controlled HIV prevention devices.

The conferences and meetings held for microbicides were organized to create translocal relationships in the global microbicide movement among donor organizations, medical and social scientists, advocates, community workers, and trial participants, facilitating the flow of drugs, devices, people, funds, and biological matter between the Global North and South. With the Global South, and particularly Africa, playing a prominent role in microbicide narratives, institutions were formed specifically around these priorities. In 2004, the African Microbicide Advocacy Group (AMAG), representing 27 African countries and a membership of 350 individuals, was founded to focus on Africa-specific interests in microbicide development: it "looks forward to a society where equity and justice prevail; and where the African woman is empowered to protect herself against HIV and AIDS; and where there is an Africa-driven agenda for more prevention options and access to information and products" (Nweneka 2007). The proliferation of microbicide organizations continues, with groups such as the International Rectal Microbicide Advocates (IRMA) network, which was established in 2005 and supports the development of rectal microbicides, potentially for gay men and also women who have anal intercourse.

In their campaigns and promotion efforts, microbicide agencies and advocates present the continuities in the discourse of women's empowerment from birth control to microbicides as relatively seamless. Historical links—fictive or otherwise—are unashamedly exploited in marketing strategies for microbicides and their funding. The GCM touts microbicides as "the most important innovation in reproductive health since the Pill." Key players in the microbicide advocacy movement express these continuities in their biographical narratives. For example, Anna Forbes (2010) writes:

> In 1972, I was 17 years old and a Planned Parenthood intern. Oral contraceptives had been available for barely a decade, and we were still 18 months away from a court decision that would legalize abortion across the US. I saw the fear and hardship of women who traveled to another state for safe abortions and the deadly horror of the illegal ones. And yet, the "old heads" in the office (as I then cavalierly regarded my elders) talked about how much more frequent this suffering had been before the pill. I saw the difference one new tool can make in women's lives.

Similarly, a GCM fundraising campaign used the figure of Katherine McCormick, a philanthropist who underwrote much of the initial development of the contraceptive pill (Bell 2003). The following news item from a 2002 GCM newsletter describes an awards dinner to celebrate Mary Ann Stein—one of the new "Mrs. McCormicks":

> "Mrs. McCormicks" are women of vision and means who have the opportunity to protect future generations from sexually transmitted infections as Katherine McCormick helped protect earlier generations from unwanted pregnancy. . . . The awards dinner reminded everyone

of the power of one woman to make a difference. . . . The international attendees were impressed by Mary Ann's enormous contribution to microbicides advocacy, and the award presentation was accompanied by the ululations of a dozen African women. As a participant from Kenya wrote to Mary Ann, "Where are the others like you? We women from Africa salute you! Your contribution could save an entire generation in Africa!" Mary Ann was inspired to see so many powerful advocates together in one place, wrestling with difficult issues, and ready to "lead us into a millennium free from fear of sexual disease."

Just like the original Mrs. McCormick, who had championed the development of the contraceptive pill during the 1950s and 1960s, the new Mrs. McCormicks were to inspire hope of discovering a method for women, particularly African women, to use against HIV.

Many microbicide narratives transcend the link with reproductive rights in the Global North by stressing the voices of women in the Global South. Contemporary accounts emphasize that microbicides did not come exclusively from within a scientific framework, but from a "grassroots" and often "African" demand for something better than a condom. Heise (2016) notes that "the demand for microbicides emerged from the voices and experiences of grassroots women who were really clear that if male condoms were the only option on offer, they would have little chance to protect themselves. Many felt that it was impossible to raise the issue of condom use with husbands and other long term partners. It was this reality that early advocates tried to highlight, drawing analogies to early efforts to help women realize their reproductive intentions." Heise (2009) recalls that the idea of a microbicide first struck her at a US Agency for International Development (USAID) meeting, when a peer educator from Uganda spoke about her experience of trying to promote condoms among women: "If the condom is all I can offer, I can't even start the discussion—but they want to get pregnant. Either you expose yourself to a disease or don't get pregnant." This reference to the microbicide industry responding to African women's demands for alternatives is a constant leitmotif. It bestows legitimacy on the technology as a scientific response to a local demand.

The voices of ordinary women are often quoted in microbicide literature to illustrate their support. In a GCM (2011) newsletter, the following quotes were featured:

I am tired of talking every day to other sex workers about condoms and not making a difference. I wish these microbicides would come so that I can just keep quiet and give them out.

If I was eligible, I would love to participate in a trial so that I can contribute to the future of my grandkids and my great grand kids.

These microbicides give me hope.

I can see the day when I hide my microbicide in my vegetable garden and when I go to pick up veggies, I can quickly put it in my vagina and go inside the house with no worries about being infected with HIV by my husband.

As can be seen throughout microbicide publications, women are portrayed as actively encouraging microbicide research and development. Heise (2009) recalls a tension between the structural and the biomedical in community consultations:

Some very brave African women stood up and said, "Look, we have listened quietly for the last two days and we understand all these political issues, but we are dying, our sisters are dying, and it cannot be framed as an either/or. We need to work on the structural issues and we need new tools."

Emphasizing the urgency of providing women with technologies they can control, advocates use the endorsement of African women to refute the criticism that biotechnology does not address the political, social, or economic dimensions of AIDS.[5]

Although it took many years to shift the opinions of HIV advocates, scientists, and donors, microbicides have become mainstream and fundable, moving from the periphery of biomedical research toward the center (Bell 2003; Heise 2009). As researchers switched with increasing ease between advocacy and science, these identities became fluid, signaling a "democratization" of medicine and technology (Bell 2003), with microbicides demonstrating the natural integration of reproductive science and virology from the Global North with the needs and demands of women from the Global South. Yet even as the microbicide movement stresses the power of science to transform women's lives positively, their messages are based on enduring assumptions about the fundamental nature of Africans, coupled with feminist notions of empowerment. While microbicides are marketed as a revolutionary technology, the narratives that underpin their popularity among advocates and researchers—black women asking for help from pharmaceuticals and (presumably white) doctors—are far more conventional and invoke familiar tropes of infested natives and the power of medical revolutions. The portrayal of African culture as a risk factor for HIV, and biomedical interventions as an effective solution, reinforces ethnic and racial boundaries through the language of science. Similar to tuberculosis catechisms, current discussions of microbicides reframe social ills, in this case gender inequality, in terms of a medical crisis. Most importantly, the solution to these pathological and pervasive behavioral patterns can be found in biotechnology. As an empowering HIV prevention method, microbicides merge the medical and social into a single disorder that is to be treated through a pharmaceutical. Medicalizing gender and race for the twenty-first century, white feminist aspirations for black women are to be realized through drugs.

# 2    Testing Hope

A potent symbol in the "war against AIDS," microbicide technology has undergone significant growth over the last three decades. As the concept of a microbicide achieved widespread acceptance, projects to develop and test this technology attracted more investors. When the GCM began in 1998 there was only $200,000 for microbicide research, but as advocates stressed its hopeful nature, interest in product development expanded rapidly. Appealing to the urgency of finding an effective microbicide, the GCM's Anna Forbes stated, "There is little doubt, that with sufficient investment, a microbicide could be available within five years. The women of the world, as well as their partners and children, desperately need and deserve more options" (Boonstra 2000). Appeals such as this succeeded in drawing in new donors. In 2002, global funding, including philanthropic, pharmaceutical, and government donations, increased by a massive 62 percent. By 2007, microbicide funding amounted to about $140 million in the United States and $226 million worldwide (HIV Vaccines and Microbicides Resource Tracking Working Group 2008). Five years later, contributions from public, philanthropic, and commercial sectors added up to a record $245 million (HIV Vaccines and Microbicides Resource Tracking Working Group 2013).

A substantial portion of this money has been devoted to randomized clinical trials. Lengthy, expensive, and involving large numbers of volunteers and staff, clinical trial research consumed almost half (46 percent) of all microbicide funding (HIV Vaccines and Microbicides Resource Tracking Working Group 2008). Several large US- and UK-based networks and programs manage trials in sub-Saharan Africa, Thailand, the United States, and South America, financed through grants from a range of governmental and nongovernmental agencies, including the NIH, USAID, DFID, the British Medical Research Council (MRC), and the Bill and Melinda Gates Foundation. This has resulted in a vast global microbicide trial network. Seven large-scale clinical microbicide trials, involving an estimated twenty thousand women participants, have taken place (Woodsong et al. 2013). These trials are the outcome of several years of in vitro testing of new drugs, small animal and primate studies to assess safety and effect, and human safety studies (phase I). Only then can "proof of concept" (phase II) and larger efficacy trials (phase III) be implemented. If these demonstrate efficacy and safety, further effectiveness and safety studies may be conducted, leading to licensure and distribution.

Clinical trials play such a large role in microbicide research and funding because it is only through this evidence-based path that a new product will be declared a success. As with other medical innovations, clinical trials are not the result of a single scientific trajectory but rather the consequence of historical, economic, and social circumstances. As new drugs were developed in the first half of the twentieth century, physicians sought a process to limit the impact of psychological factors such as the placebo effect in shaping pharmaceutical testing (Löwy 2000:50). Soon after the Second World War, placebos, randomization, double-blinding, and careful statistical analysis were combined to create the mechanisms and methods of modern trials. In recent years, the number of clinical trials and the number of people participating in them have grown dramatically thanks to the development of new drugs, as well as the increasing influence of medical rights advocacy and a burgeoning neoliberal health care environment. Despite their apparent scientific veracity, however, clinical trials have been labeled as potentially if not unavoidably unethical. Although microbicide advocates seek to empower women and prevent HIV, a certain percentage of participants must contract HIV over the course of a trial if a formulation is to be scientifically proven effective. But even as researchers argue that finding a female-controlled prophylaxis outweighs potential risks, a microbicide has yet to be licensed and released to the public.

Despite a great deal of funding and a great many trials, the scientific evidence to support the hope in microbicides is at best uncertain and at worst dubious. While over 90 percent of all HIV prevention trials are flat (Padian et al. 2010), microbicide trials have an even greater failure rate. Only one microbicide has so far been found to be partially effective in preventing HIV infection, and not a single formulation has been licensed for distribution.[1] Despite concerns about lack of efficacy, there remains faith in microbicides because each clinical trial is an exercise in creating hope: the outcomes are unknown until revealed at the end of the trial, while the mystery around the potential efficacy of the product being tested encourages confidence and opti-mism. Hope has "enormous political and economic potential" (Crapanzano 2003:8) and microbicides' appeal to a vision of women's empowerment con-tinues to drive investments. Through what DelVecchio Good (2001) terms a "political economy of hope," clinical research creates relationships between research scientists, advocates, trial participants, and funders. The continued investment in biotechnology is sustained primarily through aspirations that are engendered not "from material products with therapeutic efficacy but through the production of ideas, with potential although not yet proven therapeutic efficacy" (DelVecchio Good 2001:397). While evidence-based medicine was designed to eliminate the "unscientific" social perceptions of drugs, clinical trials have come to embody the hope of medical researchers, trial participants, and the public at large.

## THE DEVELOPMENT OF THE RANDOMIZED CLINICAL TRIAL

Like the development of medicine in general, the advent of clinical trials is often portrayed as a linear advancement toward greater knowledge and more efficacious methods. But this narrative of a progressive trajectory is derived from contemporary views and aspirations. As the methods of clinical trials change, so too do the histories (Dehue 2010:105). While the randomized clinical trial was developed only after the Second World War, there is a per-vasive tendency to trace its roots to a much earlier period. When seeking the earliest evidence of medical experimentation resembling clinical trials, many researchers and clinical trial websites point to the Bible. The Book of Daniel recounts how King Nebuchadnezzar ordered his subjects to eat a diet of meat and wine to sustain good health. When some objected to this decree, he allowed the dissenters to have a diet of water and legumes for ten days. Upon completion of the "trial," the king determined that the vegetarians appeared to be better nourished than those eating meat and allowed them to con-tinue their diet. Clinical trial historians argue that the comparative aspect of the "experiment," coupled with its impact on "public health," resembles key aspects of modern clinical trials (Bhatt 2010:6). While medicine has sought to disassociate itself from religion in many ways, the story of Nebuchadnezzar nevertheless ties medical innovation to biblical lessons.

The first controlled clinical trial of the "modern era" is credited to James Lind (1716–1794) for his work with sailors suffering from scurvy

(Bhatt 2010:7). While at sea in 1747, Lind attempted to treat twelve patients using six alternate therapies: a quart of cider per day, twenty-five drops of elixir vitriol three times a day, two spoonfuls of vinegar three times a day, sea water, two oranges and one lemon a day, and a mixture of drugs recommended by a hospital surgeon. To ensure that any changes in health were the result of the treatment and no other factors, the patients were kept together and given a standard diet. Although those consuming citrus fared the best, followed by those taking cider, Lind was reluctant to recommend citrus as a treatment because of its high cost. As a result, almost 50 years would pass before lemon juice was made a standard part of a sailor's diet in Britain (Bhatt 2010:7). Soon thereafter, lime juice was used as a substitute because it cost less. While Lind's investigation is lauded for its attempt to establish an accurate comparison, it also illustrates the critical role of economic motivations and constraints in medical research.

Despite experiments such as Lind's, almost two hundred years would elapse before true standardized research was developed, because the cornerstone of clinical trials—the assumption that under certain conditions groups of humans can be reliably compared—was largely doubted until the twentieth century. Although John Stuart Mill's *A System of Logic* (1843) outlined a scheme of comparative research methods, he nevertheless asserted that true case compatibility did not exist among humans and therefore these techniques could not be applied to actual research. Taking humans out of their context, comparing them, and then drawing conclusions that would be applied to others seemed nonsensical at the time. Because differences in race, nationality, and class were considered too great to overcome reliably, many intellectuals of the era thought medicine should focus on systematic observation rather than comparative experimentation (Dehue 2010:107). Nineteenth-century beliefs in the fundamental biological disparity of humans not only formed the bedrock of scientific racism but also effectively prohibited the development of randomized clinical trials. Consequently, it was not until scientific attitudes began to stress the similarity in human variation that comparative medical research became possible.

While changing views of human biology laid the intellectual groundwork for the development of clinical trials, technological and economic advances also played a strong role. As improvements in chemical engineering allowed a greater range of drugs to be synthesized, chemical companies saw an opportunity to diversify operations while increasing their revenue streams and began creating, marketing, and selling larger quantities of pharmaceuticals (Löwy 2000:50). Each new drug was touted as a quick cure for a range of illnesses, but the claims made by chemical companies were often based on a desire to sell their products rather than conclusive testing. Unsure of which medicines were best, doctors sought trustworthy and impartial information. Although links between medical research laboratories and the chemical industry were firmly established by the twentieth century, physicians sought to create a reliable method to evaluate new therapies transparently and objectively. But it wasn't until the outbreak of the Second World War that the urgent need for effective drugs permanently altered medical research.

Just as a desire to control colonial possessions had previously spurred tropical health research, the wartime demand for systematic drug distribution and testing prompted the creation of full-fledged clinical trials. With syphilis and gonorrhea afflicting many soldiers, conquering sexually transmitted infections became a priority for the US military (Marks 2000:100). Penicillin and streptomycin, two recently developed drugs, held the promise of treating these infections, but definitive evidence of their efficacy was elusive. In the past, these drugs would have been evaluated by independent research organizations, resulting in diverse and often contradictory reports. Then only after several years of sifting through data would a pharmaceutical have been declared efficacious. Faced with the exigencies of war, the United States could not afford to wait years while these drugs underwent independent testing.

In an effort to bring pharmaceuticals to market in record time, close government partnerships with industrial and research bodies were forged. To ensure a regular supply of drugs, the government ordered an increase in penicillin production and imposed a monopoly on its use (107). Centrally planned and coordinated studies were devised to compare large samples under similar conditions. The subsequent penicillin trials were highly controlled and many doctors disliked having to follow a standardized protocol that did not allow them to prescribe additional or alternate regimens based on their clinical experiences. Despite the goal of uniformity, variations in race, gender, and stage of disease confounded results. In addition, half of the patient sample was discarded because of incomplete data or a lack of follow-up (109). In spite of these setbacks, there was hope that a continued collaboration between government, industry, and research organizations could be perfected to yield large-scale results in a compressed period of time (Löwy 2000:54).

One of the key goals for standardization was to eliminate participant bias. Researchers suspected that the perceptions of either patients or physicians could influence reactions to treatment. Drawing from experiences with the long-standing use of dummy remedies, they feared that the power of suggestion rather than the therapy itself could be responsible for positive outcomes. These apprehensions dovetailed with the constraints of war to encourage the development of two fundamental methods of clinical trial research: placebos and blinding. Appearing in the 1800s, the word "placebo" initially denoted a treatment designed more to please than to benefit (Bhatt 2010:7). In the eighteenth and nineteenth centuries, doctors soothed their patients with placebos when there was no conventional treatment available. While Austin Flint (1863) employed a placebo in his study of treatments for rheumatic fever in 1863, it was not until the twentieth century that "placebo" began to refer to a dummy treatment in drug trials. By the 1940s, the use of placebos was accepted as a tool that promoted greater standardization in drug experimentation, but it was shortages during the war that prompted placebo-controlled trials on a wider scale. When one component of an analgesic was in limited supply, a placebo trial was conducted to determine if the component was in fact necessary (Jellinek 1946).

With the introduction of placebos came the need for a reliable method of assigning patients to a treatment arm. Initially, doctors identified "ideal specimens" and assigned them to active treatments (Marks 2000:110). However, if trials were to be truly standardized, this system had to be changed. Researchers also recognized that physicians might knowingly or unknowingly treat participants differently if their treatment status was known. The solution was to blind not only patients but also physicians. The first double-blind trial occurred in 1943 under the auspices of the MRC. During a trial to test the effects of patulin on the common cold, patients were taken into a designated room, assigned to a treatment arm by nursing staff, and given identical-looking medications (Chalmers and Clarke 2004). Rather than allocating patients based on a set of ideal characteristics, nurses alternated treatment by enrollment order.

The outcomes of the penicillin and patulin trials convinced many researchers that they were on the right track to developing an effective testing framework. Keen to refine the techniques further, they conducted a series of trials in the United States and United Kingdom to evaluate the antibiotic streptomycin as a tuberculosis treatment. In previous trials, investigators had sought to limit bias by introducing a placebo, by double-blinding, and by alternating therapies. However, there were concerns that this would not be sufficient for the streptomycin trials. Tuberculosis patients had been known to recover spontaneously; doctors thus wondered how to prove conclusively that a drug was ultimately responsible for a successful outcome (Yoshioka 1998:1221). Sir Austin Bradford Hill, an epidemiologist at the London School of Hygiene and Tropical Medicine, argued that certainty could be found through the use of statistical methods. Prior to the 1940s, statisticians and doctors had shared a "mutual indifference," but Hill was convinced that by embracing randomization, doctors could use chance to distribute factors beyond their own control or even knowledge, rendering those factors statistically inert (Marks 2000:138). Allowing statistics to work through randomization would ensure that valid comparisons could be drawn over a relatively wide range of participants (Löwy 2000:51).

Hill's vision of harnessing the power of statistics guided the MRC trials. To ground the results as firmly in objective fact as possible, patient recovery was determined through chest x-rays read by independent experts, rather than by the doctors administering treatment (Löwy 2000:51). Given that streptomycin was in short supply, researchers were able to argue that a placebo arm was both statistically and ethically justified (Bhatt 2010:8). And for the first time, patients were fully randomized. Randomization not only provided an analytic framework for the trials but also sent a clear message about the fairness of medical research in a time of limited resources. In an era when external pressure could be exerted to provide treatment to specific participants, randomization relieved clinicians of having to decide which patients were assigned a placebo, thus allowing them to evade accusations of favoritism (Yoshioka 1998:1223). The impact of these trials was profound: "For many of those of us who had been involved in the MRC streptomycin trial, randomized trials became a way of life, and provided much of the evidence upon which rational treatment policies came to be based" (Crofton 2006:533). With multiple protocols in place to replace subjectivity with probability, the modern clinical trial was born.

## ETHICS, ADVOCACY, AND NEOLIBERALISM

While the implementation of objectivized trials changed beliefs about managing data, it did not alter existing trends surrounding the treatment of research participants. Aside from concerns over how the public would view a placebo arm, there was little discussion of ethics. For Hill and others, the greatest potential harm that might result from trials was the release of a drug that was either ineffective or injurious (Marks 2000:158). An ethical trial was one that used pharmaceutical and statistical resources in an objective manner to arrive at objective conclusions. The issues of informed consent, protection of privacy, and treatment of human subjects were not viewed as critical when compared to effective trial management. Nevertheless, revelations of Nazi experimentation at the close of World War II led to the adoption of the Nuremberg Code of research ethics in 1947. Although the Nuremberg Code stressed the importance of obtaining voluntary informed consent from all research subjects, these guidelines were not always met. Physicians and researchers argued that their research, while not always following the new ethical guidelines, was vastly different from the Nazi experiments (Fisher 2008:24). Nazi research was portrayed as negative because of its perceived ideological and state-driven motivation. In contrast, studies in the United States were cast positively as independent and apolitical. Consequently, trial coordinators argued that informed consent and voluntary participation could be ignored if scientifically warranted.

Histories recounting clinical trials as a triumphant series of scientific and methodological breakthroughs often fail to note that many experiments and medical procedures were performed on stigmatized, minority, and vulnerable populations. Perhaps the most infamous example is the Tuskegee syphilis experiment. Conducted from 1932 to 1972 with funding from the Public Health Service, the study enrolled 600 impoverished male African American sharecroppers, 399 of whom had contracted syphilis. Uninformed that they were enrolled in a research project, these individuals were told that they were receiving free medical care for "bad blood." However, participants were given only placebos, as the study sought to monitor the development and long-term effects of syphilis. Although it was subsequently discovered that penicillin was an effective cure for syphilis, this knowledge was withheld from the participants, and effective treatment was not provided to them (Jones 1993). Tuskegee was not an isolated event.

Throughout the United States, nonconsenting research subjects were drawn from marginalized groups and exposed to hazardous and harmful testing. When medical researchers designed the first clinical trials in the 1940s to evaluate the effectiveness of sulfa drugs in treating sexually acquired infections, they argued that the most effective way to procure the required population was by infecting prison inmates. After extensive deliberations, the trial was approved, only to be halted once it was discovered that the procedure for inflicting gonorrhea was unreliable (Marks 2000:105). Prisoners remained a popular source of human subjects and it has been estimated that 90 percent of drugs licensed prior to the 1970s were assessed in these populations (Harkness 1996; Petryna 2006:38). Residents of other institutions such as orphanages and psychiatric facilities were also used for pharmaceutical testing. During the 1960s, youths from the Willowbrook State School for Retarded Children were exposed to hepatitis to gauge the effectiveness of gamma globulin. Researchers argued that actively infecting the children was the only way to ensure the standardization and controlled conditions necessary for reliable results (Fisher 2008:22). Minority populations were also targeted. Seeking information regarding the precise toxicity of radiation, the Public Health Service conducted a ten-year study from the 1940s to 1950s in which Navajo uranium miners were denied protective gear to understand how quickly exposure would lead to death (ibid.).

While investigators continued to defend their research ethics, a series of highly publicized cases led to greater governmental control and oversight. In 1966, Dr. Henry Beecher described 22 examples of unethical research, and a few years later the details of the Tuskegee syphilis study made headlines (Harkness et al. 2001). In response, the World Medical Association drafted the Declaration of Helsinki (1964), which expanded the ten principles of the Nuremberg Code to specifically address clinical research. Although the declaration is not a legally binding document, it has nevertheless been revised to clarify changing practices in medical research. In the United States, greater ethical regulation of medical research occurred through the National Research Act of 1974 and Belmont Report of 1979. The latter stressed the importance of informed consent while simultaneously weighing participant risks against societal benefits. More recently, in response to the rise of clinical trials worldwide, the ICH (International Conference on Harmonisation of Technical Requirements for Registration of Pharmaceuticals for Human Use) released *Guideline for Good Clinical Practice* (1996), a set of global standards for individual governments to model their medical research policies on.

Despite the proliferation of documents, policies, and regulations regarding the treatment of human subjects in medical research, ethics remain flexible in practice. Noting the frequency with which guidelines are reformulated, Adriana Petryna (2006:46) characterizes ethics regulations as "workable documents" imbued with variability. Medical researchers and industry professionals consulted throughout the drafting of standards have claimed that restrictions would stifle development and slow drugs to market (Fisher 2008:29). As a result, while recommendations ostensibly protect patient welfare, they nevertheless allow researchers to deviate from these ideals in particular circumstances, such as medical crises or international research. Ongoing debates regarding the variability of ethical standards have been impacted by two seemingly contrasting trends: advocacy and neoliberalism. On one hand, the need to develop drugs quickly to address the rise of life-threatening illnesses has created medical advocacy groups concerned with protecting the well-being of patients, while on the other, pharmaceutical companies and medical research organizations have become increasingly focused on the profitability of new drugs and the ability to market them successfully.

Beginning in the 1970s, clinical trials shifted from being conceived primarily as statistical tools to determine efficacy to an embodiment of hope and profit. As cancer afflicted Americans in record numbers, new pharmaceuticals were seen as the most effective treatment. Given the rapidity with which some cancers spread, there was an urgency to test drugs as quickly as possible. Furthermore, the high mortality rate of many cancers led patients to adopt an attitude that they had little to lose from agreeing to radical and risky procedures. As ever-greater numbers of participants were recruited into cancer trials, researchers regularly deviated from approved standards. Studies increasingly lacked placebo arms or randomization, and experimentation on "desperate" patients was commonplace (Löwy 2000:61–62). Over time, oncology became oriented toward medical research, and clinical trials were transformed into routine therapy. Examining autologous bone-marrow transplants for metastatic breast cancer, Mary-Jo DelVecchio Good (2007) asserts that despite initially lackluster results, oncologists encouraged this procedure to the extent that the experimental became normalized. This process was facilitated by a medical imaginary, which portrays biomedicine as invariably producing life-saving drugs through research. The hope that an experimental drug engenders, rather than its statistical effectiveness, facilitates its prescription by doctors and adoption by patients. Along with the potential of effectiveness comes not just a flow of human subjects but also financial investment. DelVecchio Good writes, "The biotechnical embrace creates a popular culture that is enamored with the biology of hope, attracting venture capital that continues even in the face of contemporary constraints to generate new treatment modalities" (377). Embraced by the optimistic discourse of medicine, clinical trials have moved from standardized statistical tools to vehicles embodying the promise of health.

While cancer research routinized clinical trials, the early quest for AIDS treatments further altered attitudes toward experimental drugs. Ascribing the lack of an effective treatment for HIV to an overly lengthy and complex FDA approval process, advocates assumed an increasingly active role in medical dialogues and interventions surrounding HIV (Löwy 2000:53). Born out of the gay rights movement, this lobby did not trust the medical establishment to treat gay men responsibly, given that doctors and psychologists had historically labeled them as pathological. Drawing from organizations and resources devoted to gay activism, and modeling their efforts after earlier cancer campaigns, advocates pushed for larger trials with less restrictive recruitment in an attempt to speed drugs to market, challenging the monopoly on drug testing that was shared by the government, pharmaceutical producers, statisticians, and physicians. Examining the profound effects of AIDS advocacy, Steven Epstein (1995:409) notes "that activist movements, through amassing different forms of credibility, can in certain circumstances become genuine participants in the construction of scientific knowledge—that they can (within definite limits) effect changes both in the epistemic practices of biomedical research and in the therapeutic techniques of medical care." Circumventing rigid institutional testing, "heroic" patients took parallel therapies and organized unofficial trials (Löwy 2000:63). Responding to this pressure and declaring HIV an emergency, the US government fast-tracked HIV drug research. Rather than accepting roles as passive subjects, people with HIV and AIDS actively guided the medical research process by engaging in public dialogue as well as participating in clinical trials.

With the release of AZT, the first highly effective antiretroviral therapy, independent and parallel testing occurred far less frequently. By the end of the 1990s, the era of informal patient-oriented trials had ended, and all of the major HIV drugs were produced by large multinational companies. Furthermore, as rates of HIV in sub-Saharan Africa exceeded those of North American and European nations, drug trials were shifted offshore. Lacking the input of strong local advocates, AIDS trials in developing nations were once again primarily conceptualized in terms of statistics. With the seeming reintroduction of carefully controlled samples, the use of a placebo, which had fallen out of use in some HIV trials, was again encouraged in international settings. When researchers began testing the ability of a short course of AZT to prevent mother-to-child HIV transmission in Uganda, South Africa, Tanzania, Côte d'Ivoire, Burkina Faso, and Thailand, a placebo was introduced despite data showing that a full course of AZT was effective. Subsequently, the trial was criticized—and in some cases compared to Tuskegee—for using a placebo instead of the proven therapy as a baseline for statistical comparison (Petryna 2006:43). Members of the NIH and the Centers for Disease Control, the institutions that had authorized and funded the trial, defended their protocol, arguing that a placebo arm had been necessary on scientific grounds as "it offers more definitive answers and a clearer view of side effects" (Varmus and Satcher 1997:1005). Furthermore, they reasoned that participants would not have had access to a full course of AZT because of its high cost, and therefore assigning them to the placebo arm had not been equivalent to denying treatment. Despite these justifications, the short-course trial was widely deemed unethical, and additional guidelines for trials have been adopted as a result.[2]

In recent years, international trials have come under closer scrutiny in part because the ethical standards of the United States or European nations are often not followed as diligently when research is conducted abroad. Despite global guidelines for human subject participation, medical researchers argue for ethical variability when conducting trials in non-Western nations, noting that cultural norms can make it necessary to ignore or alter guidelines governing the treatment of participants (Petryna 2006). As a result, there has been a tendency to label international trials as fundamentally exploitative or even neocolonial (Nundy and Gulhati 2005). Critics note that a great many of these trials are conducted among impoverished and undereducated populations in countries with struggling public health care systems, so even when the principle of informed consent is strictly followed, the health care and remuneration offered by trials unduly motivate participants to overlook any potential risks involved (Fisher 2008). Furthermore, guidelines focusing on individuals and individual consent fail to recognize and adjust for the structural factors that make possible the disadvantaged populations who have historically been the primary participants in medical research (Petryna 2005).

Such structural factors have become more visible as neoliberalism increasingly impacts medical practice. Instead of supporting a health care system controlled and regulated through the state and its apparatus, medical neoliberalism encourages private corporations, pharmaceutical companies, and medical treatment facilities to market their services directly to patients, who are then recast as consumers (Fisher 2008:14). No longer a right to be enjoyed by all citizens, medical care becomes an amenity provided to those who can afford it. As a result, many pharmaceuticals are developed outside of the medical crisis paradigm of cancer and HIV. Although cancer trials continue to be the most prevalent in the United States, there has been a significant rise in trials for chronic and preventable conditions (6). With so many new drugs being developed, researchers require an ever-growing number of participants who are healthy or symptom-free. Trial organizers face difficulties in recruiting, and the resultant delays are thought not only to slow the time to market but also limit profitability. In an effort to facilitate drug testing, many aspects of the research process are becoming outsourced and trials are shifting from academic medical institutions to corporate firms.

There is now a clinical trial industry that consists of for-profit institutional review boards (IRBs), clinical trial advertising agencies, and contract research organizations (CROs), companies specializing in tasks such as participant recruitment, data management, preclinical research, and biologic assay development. Paralleling direct-to-consumer advertising of drugs, CROs market trials through television commercials, newspaper ads, and websites. Far more than just tools to increase recruitment, these messages create and reinforce notions regarding the use of medicine in everyday life, with trial participation regularly portrayed as a responsible and individual choice that will assist the development of life-enhancing therapies. This narrative further pharmaceuticalizes well-being. With greater numbers of healthy individuals taking drugs through trials, pharmaceutical use has become part of a daily routine (Dumit 2012). Furthermore, the availability of trials obfuscates economic inequality and the rising cost of health care. Many CROs efficiently advertise trials as medical care for the uninsured, making trials the "responsible choice" in a neoliberal system (Fisher 2008:17). With low-paying service jobs becoming the norm in many parts of the United States, the number of individuals enrolling in trials as a primary form of income— professional guinea pigs—has grown (Abadie 2010:135). The focus on the care provided by trials recasts them as medical opportunities rather than a last resort for low-wage earners.

Given these trends, there has been a tendency to assume that most clinical trials are under the complete control of Western corporations, with participants who are relatively powerless and thus cannot direct the protocols or outcomes of these projects. However, the realities behind clinical trials are far more complex. It is more productive to assess trials as processes through which private industry and the state wield varying degrees of social, political, and economic capital. Although pharmaceutical corporations often do engineer and conduct trials, activists and patient advocates press them for equity in the trials' implementation. Furthermore, through regulation and in some cases funding, the state also constrains the parameters of clinical trials. Finally, human subjects themselves impact trials and their results through their participation or lack thereof. The multilayered interactions that shape trials, as well as contrasting views of clinical research ethics, can be witnessed in attempts to bring an efficacious microbicide to market.

## THE MICROBICIDE TRIALS

The rise and continuing prevalence of microbicide trials simultaneously differ from and resemble recent developments in clinical trials across the board. While trials generally have become increasingly controlled by pharmaceutical companies seeking profit, this has not occurred in microbicide research. Microbicide trialists acknowledge that there will be little profit to be made in the marketing and selling of any product proven to be effective, as the women who would potentially use microbicides would be unable to afford an expensive pharmaceutical. Consequently, most of the trials are coordinated from within academic research institutes or units attached to academic departments, and funded through state research bodies such as medical research councils, the NIH, and the DFID. Monies are not only drawn from public tax funds but also international donors and philanthropic organizations such as the Bill and Melinda Gates Foundation. Given their reliance on these funds, microbicide trials incur lower overall costs per patient than commercial trials, in part because the compounds being tested are made available at low or no cost. Furthermore, because microbicides are envisioned as a technology to aid poor women in the developing world, their testing has been driven by advocates keen to promote female autonomy and empowerment. In line with this model, trialists strive to consult with local communities and the women who may participate.

Regardless of advocacy and donor-driven models, the gold standard for microbicide trials remains statistical verification through the use of a placebo. Participants are randomized to either a gel containing the active product or a placebo gel, both of which resemble a vaginal lubricant. Great care must be taken to ensure that the placebo gel has minimal effect on the flora of the vaginal tract and that it is virtually indistinguishable from the active gel. To determine the initial safety of the product, phase I trials are often held in Europe or North America. Subsequent trials to determine dosage (phase II) and efficacy (phase III) are conducted in Asia and Africa because of the high prevalence of HIV in these settings. To confirm that the trial is adequately powered statistically (to demonstrate that an effect of the drug being tested is in fact caused by the drug rather than other factors), phase III trials require large cohorts of participants and take into consideration HIV prevalence rates, condom use, product adherence rates, possible attrition from the trial, and suspension of product use when, for example, a participant becomes pregnant. The sheer size of the trials—regularly enrolling several thousand women—necessitates the involvement of multiple clinic sites, often in different countries, and even on different continents, to generate a sufficient number of participants.

But despite their goal of fostering women's and patient rights, microbicide trials continue to be confronted with significant ethical issues. Throughout sub-Saharan Africa, communities ask why researchers invariably seem to test their innovative pharmaceuticals on poor black women. While HIV prevalence rates are often cited in response, the reality is that a microbicide can be proven effective only if a statistically significant number of women on the trial contract HIV. The necessity of seroconversion creates an unresolved conflict between the humanitarian and statistical goals of microbicide trials. Although microbicide research and development has been strongly influenced by advocates and others intent on saving the lives of African women, they nonetheless acknowledge that the only way to achieve this goal is through the exposure of women to HIV. Tensions between the hope of finding an efficacious microbicide and the risk posed to poor black women have been present since microbicide trials first began in the late 1980s.

To date, three generations of microbicides have been tested through the first three trial phases (see fig. 2). The initial hope for microbicides came from already registered spermicides that had been available as over-the-counter contraceptives in North America and Europe since the 1950s. Early in vitro testing showed that in addition to acting against semen, these

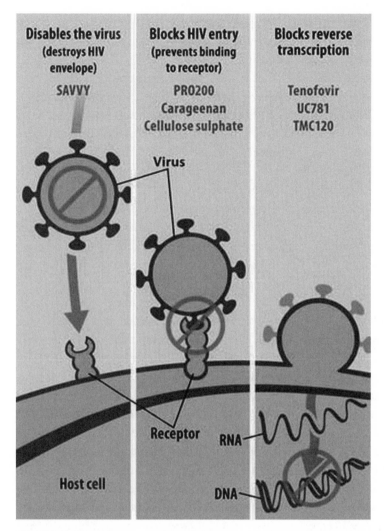

**FIGURE 2.** Site of action of candidate microbicides. Graphic by Giovanni Maki, from Jonathan Weber, Kamal Desai, and Janet Darbyshire, "The Development of Vaginal Microbicides for the Prevention of HIV Transmission." *PLoS Medicine* 2, no. 5 (2005.): e142.

detergents or surfactants affected HIV and other sexually transmitted infections by disrupting the membranes of microbial pathogens (Lederman et al. 2006). Subsequently, several studies were conducted to assess the safety of using various types of spermicides in different formulations, but these results were not always favorable. A 1992 trial by the Institute of Tropical Medicine

(Antwerp, Belgium), testing menfegol foaming tablets among 125 prostitutes in Senegal over a 14-day period, was terminated early after women experienced high rates of vaginal lesions (Goeman et al. 1995).[3]

The focus then shifted to COL-1492, a gel containing nonoxynol-9, an over-the-counter spermicide. Researchers worried that repeated use of N-9 in the high dosages found to combat HIV in vitro could lead to epithelial disruptions, which would actually increase the risk of contracting the virus. Safety assessments of COL-1492 after phase II showed that although epithelial lesions had been found, they had occurred in less than 3 percent of the trial population in both the placebo and active arms. With safety no longer a concern, COL-1492 became the first gel containing N-9 to progress to a phase III trial. The subsequent four-year trial was sponsored by UNAIDS and enrolled female sex workers from four countries: Benin, Côte d'Ivoire, South Africa, and Thailand. In June 2000, the study findings revealed that 449 women randomly allocated to the active N-9 gel were 50 percent more likely to become infected with HIV. Although it was never confirmed, this was assumed to be the result of epithelial lesions among women using the gel.

In her analyses of the ethical implications of the trial, one of the lead investigators at a South African site, Gita Ramjee, draws attention to the limited understanding that participants had of informed consent, the difficulties participants experienced in using condoms, and the standard of care that excluded treatment for women who seroconverted during the trial (Ramjee 2007; Ramjee et al. 2000). However, a critical issue that Ramjee does not fully explore is the targeting of sex workers for experimental trials. It was common for early phase II and III trials to recruit subjects from populations of sex workers, where a higher than average HIV incidence, of approximately 2.5 percent per year, was assumed (van de Wijgert and Jones 2006). Sex workers are an ideal group because the higher potential incidence of HIV reduced the size of the population required to observe effects of the candidate microbicide. However, the COL-1492 trial disregarded the behaviors of this population. Although several safety studies had been undertaken prior to the phase III trial, these did not factor in the high rates of sexual activity and therefore the multiple gel use on an average day by sex workers. The more the gel was used, the greater its potential toxicity. While sex workers were an ideal population for trial purposes because of their repeated exposure to HIV, the frequency of sexual contacts increased the negative side effects of the gel.[4] Another important aspect that was not factored into the design of the trial was the high prevalence of anal sex among sex workers, which may have also been a source of HIV infection (Ramjee and Karim 1998). Given these findings, COL-1492 researchers have been criticized for lacking foresight in taking N-9 to trial (Grant et al. 2008). A commentator on the UN-moderated GENDER-AIDS e-mail network noted that "the drawbacks to N-9 are well known but that had to be balanced against its fast track possibilities" (quoted in Tallis 2012:116). While the possibility of quickly releasing an effective microbicide motivated researchers to move forward with the N-9 trial, it seems to have also led trialists to overlook the inherent risks associated with the drug.

The COL-1492 trial damaged the reputation of microbicides and had far-reaching implications for the field. Alliance for Microbicide Development founder Polly Harrison remarked, "We were stunned by the results, didn't know how to handle them, and for a field just getting itself organized, they were traumatic" (Harrison 2011:2). Others described the trial outcomes as a "huge setback" (Ramjee et al. 2007), and some more critically as "a scandal" (Salyer 2001). In response to the outcomes of the trial, and the alleged inaction by the scientific community, the South Africa-based Gender AIDS Forum (GAF) launched a campaign entitled "Where Are the N-9 Women," highlighting the need to compensate and treat women who had become infected during their enrollment in the trial. Six years after the trial results were made public, a consultative meeting between representatives from the WHO, the GAF, the AMAG, and the GCM was held to discuss what went wrong and what to do going forward. The scientists present at the meeting acknowledged culpability, and a fund was established to provide compensation for the women who were affected. However, very few of the original trial participants could be found and for many it was too late (Tallis 2012). While some concern was expressed for the participants of the trial, the microbicide ideal remained relatively unchallenged. David Salyer (2001) was one of only a few researchers to dispute the promise of microbicides publicly, labeling N-9 as "snake oil," "the product of junk science," and the "Frankenstein monster of laboratory lubes."

After 13 trials undertaken since 1988, the future of N-9 as an HIV prevention compound ended in 2001 (Wilkinson et al. 2002). At a WHO meeting in Geneva, it was concluded that N-9 should not be promoted for HIV or STI prevention; it could be used as a contraceptive, but only among "low risk" women whose exposure to HIV and use of N-9 is likely to be limited

(Wilkinson 2002b). In a review of the N-9 trials conducted, the authors concluded that there was "little, if any, role for N-9 as an HIV and STI prophylactic, since there is no evidence of benefit, and some concern about harm" (Wilkinson et al. 2002:617). Given the results of the trials, some AIDS activists in the United States were even calling for a complete ban of the chemical and to remove it from the coating on condoms (Fleming 2000).

In the years that followed, microbicide trials continued to have disappointing outcomes, dampening the initial enthusiasm. Further damage to the field came by way of "folk" microbicides, such as lemon and lime juice (Lederman et al. 2006). Safety studies showed that high dosages of the citrus juices could have serious side effects, including penile and vaginal lesions, potentially increasing the possibility of HIV infection. As a result, the GCM issued warnings against using lemon juice to prevent HIV (GCM 2006). Despite these setbacks, most commentators agreed that there was a need to continue pursuing the development of a female-controlled topical gel to prevent HIV infection.

By the mid-2000s, the second generation of microbicides was being developed and tested, including the active agents of Carraguard, PRO 2000/5, and cellulose sulphate. These microbicides were based around polyanion inhibitors that target viral entry by "coating the viral envelope and masking structures necessary for attachment to the cell surface and therefore entry into the cell" (Lederman et al. 2006:375). These microbicides had two clear advantages: they were not systemically absorbed into the blood and organs, and they could feasibly be distributed through nonclinical settings, like the male and female condom (Omar and Bergeron 2011). When tested in animal and laboratory studies, second-generation compounds appeared to be more effective and less toxic than N-9 (Ramjee et al. 2010). As formulated by the Population Council, Carraguard employed the active ingredient carrageenan, which is made from a red seaweed that grows along the coasts of Nova Scotia and Chile and is the same substance used as a thickening agent in ice cream and toothpaste (BBC News 2002).[5] Having established its safety for vaginal application, the Population Council ran a phase III trial from 2004 to 2007, in Durban, Johannesburg, and Cape Town. This trial supported earlier findings that the product was safe to use, but it also showed that Carraguard had no significant impact on HIV acquisition. Although fewer HIV infections were recorded for the Carraguard group than the placebo arm, the difference was not significant enough to establish efficacy

(Skoler-Karpoff et al. 2008).[6] Nevertheless, that the product was found safe to use was regarded as a major achievement after the failure of N-9.

The other major microbicide tested during this period was cellulose sulphate (CS) a polyanionic cotton derivative produced by Polydex Pharmaceuticals Limited, in Toronto, Canada (Ramjee et al. 2010). Following the same path as those for earlier products, initial animal studies and in vitro tests showed that CS was effective in preventing HIV acquisition, and phase I and II trials established its safety for use in healthy humans. A phase III trial sponsored by the US-based not-for-profit organization Contraception Research and Development (CONRAD) was undertaken in Uganda, South Africa, and Benin, while Family Health International (now FHI 360) held a similar trial in Nigeria. After one year, the data safety and monitoring committee decided that there was sufficient evidence to conclude that women on the active arm of the trial were at greater risk of HIV infection. The CONRAD trial was halted immediately, and FHI ended its trial as a "precautionary measure." In their press statement, Polydex CEO George G. Usher and lead investigator Lut Van Damme both expressed disappointment and surprise, given that the gel had passed through eleven safety and contraceptive trials with more than five hundred participants prior to the phase III stage of testing (Polydex 2007). Other microbicide researchers were similarly frustrated with the results, noting the care the researchers had for the trial participants. Zeda Rosenberg (2007), CEO of International Partnership for Microbicides (IPM), drew attention to the "true heroes" of these trials— namely, the female participants—adding that investors had halted the trial quickly out of concern for the well-being of these women. The tenor of this and other responses indicates that the negative repercussions from the earlier N-9 trial were still being felt. One commentator remarked, "It is a sign of the state of the field that there were sighs of relief when it became clear that Carraguard had not enhanced HIV-1 transmission rates, for this was the apparent outcome of the efficacy trial of Ushercell (cellulose sulfate), yet another polyanion, last year" (Grant et al. 2008). With the end of the CS trials, microbicide research became subject to much greater public and governmental scrutiny.

While microbicide researchers note that their trials employ a community-driven model and seek to empower poor black women, and are thus unlike those of large pharmaceutical companies, they have elicited similar criticism. Throughout the testing of second-generation microbicides, popular narratives characterized these trials as exploiting vulnerable, impoverished women, while pharmaceutical research was cast as a profiteering self-interested foreign imposition. As with other HIV prevention trials conducted in developing countries, these perspectives were echoed in the local South African media (Mack et al. 2010). The closure of the CS trial was highly publicized and attracted a great deal of negative press. In an article in South African daily newspaper *City Press*, journalist Wonder Hlongwa (2007b) directly connects foreign research interests to high HIV rates in Africa and clinical trials: "Hundreds of women in South Africa, Benin, Nigeria, Uganda, and India, who are being used as human guinea pigs in the US-funded research on HIV prevention, are feared to have contracted the virus during the course of the trials." The use of the phrase "guinea pig" creates a potent link between the clinical trial and a discourse of global exploitation by comparing participants to animals (Mack et al. 2010). Other coverage was more explicit in asserting that trialists viewed participants as animals to be abused. For example, a reporter for the *Sowetan* declared that the reason why trials are conducted on black people is "because it is assumed that blacks cannot control themselves, so we make them cut pieces of their flesh and insert gels in their bodies instead of education, prevention, treatment and real empowerment. Blacks are treated as one would treat an animal" (Mngxitama 2010). These media reports had consequences for the trials. Hlongwa followed his initial story with a personal attack on Gita Ramjee, the lead scientist involved in the MRC's Durban site of the CS trial.[7] He insinuated that Ramjee had committed to too many clinical trials because she was motivated solely by funding (Hlongwa 2007a).

The South African government, which had been previously disinterested in microbicide research, became more and more involved. Echoing beliefs that stressed the harmful and exploitative nature of trials, President Thabo Mbeki commented, "Our people are being used as guinea pigs and conned into using dangerous and toxic drugs" (quoted in Hoad 2005:104). As the president questioned the morality of trials, Health Minister Manto Tshabalala-Msimang met with the lead investigators of the CS trial and announced that all microbicide trials in South Africa would be examined to determine if unethical conduct was occurring (Ramjee et al. 2007). In her official statement, Tshabala-Msimang said, "While we support innovation through health research, the government of South Africa is determined to ensure that the health of our people is not compromised in the process" (quoted in IRIN 2007). This led to a temporary cessation of all microbicide trials enrolling participants at the time. Meanwhile, Peggy Nkoyeni, the KwaZulu-Natal Department of Health minister, led an inquiry into alleged misconduct in microbicide trials, but the findings were never made public. At the same time that these probes into microbicide trials were being held, Mbeki, Tshabalala-Msimang, and Nkoyeni made public statements expressing opposition to many commonly held beliefs of AIDS researchers. The president and ministers denied that HIV caused AIDS and suggested that antiretroviral therapy was not an essential treatment (Fassin 2007; Nattrass 2007). Mbeki blocked the provision of ARV treatments such as nevirapine to HIV-positive mothers, portraying the drugs as "biological warfare of the apartheid era." Meanwhile, Tshabalala-Msimang argued that garlic and lemons could be used to treat HIV and felt that African remedies should not be "bogged down in clinical trials" (BBC News 2008). While often viewed by critics and AIDS activists as the result of ignorance, statements such as those of Mbeki and Tshabalala-Msimang are born out of a growing distrust of the North, a desire to promote what are believed to be African traditions, and the inability of trialists to address objections to clinical research comprehensively.

Faced with increasing government scrutiny and suspicion, microbicide trialists attempted to dispel what they viewed as misconceptions regarding clinical research. They pointed out that results exonerating trial administrators of wrongdoing were never publicized. Furthermore, trialists noted that journalists and government investors rarely spoke with trial participants and never consulted the IRBs that had granted clearance to the trials. Although trial administrators became more adept at speaking to the government and preparing press talking points, the public remained skeptical. During consultative meetings with local communities in KwaZulu-Natal, the leaders of the CS trial were confronted with questions about the ethical conduct of their research: Why did the trial ask "innocent women to sleep with HIV-positive men"? Was it true "that the gel increased the risk of HIV infection among innocent women?" "Why did researchers expose poor black women to the infected gel?" And how did "researchers explain the study to illiterate women?" (quoted in Ramjee et al. 2007:1170). Disregarding the highly emotive narratives of exploitation and harm evoked by phrases such as "innocent women" and "poor black women," the researchers reiterated the importance of community education about the clinical trial process and advocated changing the way in which trial results were reported in local presses (ibid.).

These recommendations failed to deal effectively with the underlying issue, that of the disproportionate vulnerabilities of black South Africans to HIV infection and the emotions surrounding this.

In some ways, the problems encountered by microbicide trials, particularly those testing N-9 and CS, were a result of hope. As with the earlier cancer and HIV treatments, researchers felt the health crisis was justification enough for moving quickly and with less oversight. Leading scientists declared, "What we cannot do is wait. The need for effective HIV prevention methods is too great" (Mellors et al. 2008). Consequently, the many scientific and operational challenges facing microbicide research and development were often overlooked in favor of a can-do attitude. The urgent desire to develop female-controlled technologies encouraged researchers to fast-track drugs, testing them on large numbers of women in the field as soon as possible. Given this sense of urgency, a competitive spirit dominated product development, resulting in duplication and resources wastage (Grant et al. 2008). As insufficient attention was paid to creating a single compound with demonstrated effectiveness and safety, several experimental microbicides were simultaneously released into the field at one time. This in turn led to numerous trials that all ended with disappointing results. Despite the costs, scandals, and frequent setbacks, the hope for developing an effective microbicide continued unabated. Indeed, Lut Van Damme, a leading scientist in four unsuccessful trials, was awarded the FHI 360 Lifetime Achievement Award in 2012 (FHI 360 2012). Researchers and advocates continued to assume that the first effective microbicide was just a trial away.

## THE MICROBICIDES DEVELOPMENT PROGRAMME 301

In 2004, the Microbicides Development Programme (MDP) began researching PRO 2000/5, a polymer gel to be inserted vaginally, with a disposable applicator. Managed through the MRC Clinical Trials Unit and Imperial College at St. Mary's Hospital, the MDP was a public-private partnership established between 16 UK, US, and African institutions, including university-based research entities, pharmaceutical companies, and donor organizations. Phase I trials established the safety and tolerability of a 0.5 percent dose of PRO 2000/5 among low-risk, sexually abstinent women. Subsequently, a phase IIb trial (HPTN 035) followed 3,101 enrolled women for an average of 20 months and demonstrated that PRO 2000/5 produced a 30 percent (albeit statistically insignificant) reduction in the HIV infection rate (Karim et al. 2011). Although the MDP301 had already begun when the HPTN 035 results were made public, they contributed to the general hope for a positive result from the MDP301 and sustained enthusiasm for the new trial. Imbued with optimism, the MDP301 sought to improve the lives of African women through advocacy and science. However, throughout the trial there was a constant tension between the protocols of evidence-based medicine and the desire to effect social change.

Unlike many other microbicide trials at the time, the MDP301 was unusually large: over twenty thousand women were screened, with more than nine thousand eventually completing the trial.[8] Participants were enrolled at thirteen clinics, which were managed by six research centers across Africa: three in South Africa, one in Tanzania, one in Uganda, and one in Zambia. This required a massive investment of funds, with the trial costing an estimated £40 million ($67 million). Monies were sourced from the DFID, with assistance from the European and Developing Countries Clinical Trials Program (EDCTP) and the International Partnership for Microbicides (IPM).[9] While the MDP301 was expensive compared to other smaller microbicide trials, the overall cost per patient was ten times cheaper than that of a commercial pharmaceutical trial (Advantage Business Media 2006). Part of the reason for the reduced cost was a deal with Indevus Technologies, a small unclassified pharmaceutical company located in Lexington, Massachusetts. PRO 2000/5 would be supplied for free to the MDP301 with the understanding that if the drug proved to be effective, Indevus would market PRO 2000/5 at a low cost to developing countries.[10]

To be eligible for enrollment, women had to be sexually active, HIV negative, and not pregnant (Nunn et al. 2009).[11] Potential participants were told that the gel was as yet unproven and that, as the only reliable method of preventing HIV acquisition, condoms should be used simultaneously with the gel. Randomized to one of three gel arms—2 percent PRO 2000/5, 0.5 percent PRO 2000/5, or placebo—participants were instructed to insert the gel no more than one hour prior to intercourse. Each participant was initially given a one-month supply: 40 gels, plus an extra 20 in case they ran short. For the duration of their 52-week enrollment, participants completed monthly visits to return unused gels and used applicators, to receive new gels for the coming month, and to receive pregnancy and HIV tests. Once every three months, they had a "long visit," during which additional questionnaires were administered. These assessed their condom use, adherence to instructions for using the gel, vaginal cleansing and insertion practices, and relationships with partners. To assist the women in answering questions during the interviews with clinic nurses, trial coordinators instructed participants to keep aide-mémoires or coital diaries. The women were to record details about their sexual behaviors (noting whether they engaged in vaginal or anal sex), their sex partners, the number of "rounds" during each sexual encounter, as well as their condom and gel use.

While the MDP301 protocol was designed to control the process of recruitment, enrollment, data collection, and clinical procedures for all sites, there was a certain level of flexibility that allowed different sites to shape the process in unique ways, recognizing the importance of local dynamics in influencing trial design. In Uganda, the MDP301 recruited serodiscordant couples (an HIV-positive male partner with a negative female partner; Abaasa et al. 2013), while in Tanzania recruitment focused on HIV-negative but high-risk women who worked in "recreational occupations," such as selling cooked food in bars and hotels (Lees et al. 2009). At the sites in Tanzania and Uganda, participants were also drawn from a younger age group (16 years or older) in comparison to the sites in Zambia and South Africa, where because of legislation governing the participation of adolescents in clinical trials, recruitment was restricted to women 18 years or older. As recruitment was community-based and not restricted to public health clinics, the MDP301 established a community component to foster engagement between the research clinics and the local populations. Emphasis was placed on ensuring "that local concerns were understood and addressed by trial teams, that community values and practices were respected, and that messages from the clinic were properly conveyed" (MDP 2009b). Consequently, significant efforts and funds were directed toward recruitment teams and social engagement activities to promote enrollment in the trial. Each site employed a liaison officer who was responsible for identifying local structures, hosting activities in the local area to raise awareness about the trial, and developing mechanisms for engagement.

A distinctive feature of the MDP301 was the inclusion of a significant social science component throughout the duration of the trial. Although previous trials had incorporated some element of the social sciences, these were limited in scope, and research questions had been confined to exploring cultural acceptability, drawing mainly on market research methodologies focusing on tactile experiences and smell (Bentley et al. 2004; Mehendale et al. 2012). The MDP301 social science component had a much wider goal and sought to understand the social dimensions of acceptability, in part by examining the effects of the gel on women's sexual health. In addition, the social scientists wanted to validate clinical data on sexual behaviors, including condom use, precoital use of the gel, and vaginal washing practices. A sub-sample of approximately 10 percent of the total trial population was enrolled into the social science study. A social science staff member interviewed each consenting participant at 4, 24, and 52 weeks after their initial enrollment. The aim was to provide a method of "triangulating" the data and confirming information gained through clinical interviews (Pool et al. 2010), such as number of sexual partners. The social science component was seen as an important source of data should there be doubts about the trial results. At each site, a social science research team consisting of interviewers and a senior social scientist conducted in-depth interviews, carried out focus groups, and undertook ethnographic research in MDP301 clinics and throughout the local community.

The inclusion of the social science component reflected the MDP301's emphasis on relating local knowledge to global clinical trial procedures. Its London personnel kept in touch with staff at the sites by using telephone conferencing, while face-to-face meetings were held at different sites on an annual basis.[12] Delegations from the United Kingdom interacted with local researchers and were able to view firsthand the operations of the trial. Meanwhile, local community members were offered opportunities to travel to conferences and meetings in other countries. Mindful that international trials were often critiqued as exploitative neocolonial projects, MDP officials in London sought to encourage and support intellectual and infrastructural advances at local trial sites. At the Johannesburg site, a new clinic space was fashioned from a refurbished building on the grounds of Chris Hani Baragwanath Hospital while temporary offices were constructed in the yard of a local gynecology practice, which would later be donated to the community. In seeking to shift money from the Global North to the Global South in an ethical and locally appropriate way, the MDP301 relied not only on the language of evidence-based medicine but also that of development.

Coopting the development narrative and situating local clinical research sites within a global medical and economic network, the MDP301 administrators sought to address what they saw as persistent disadvantages through medical intervention. The MDP301 was simultaneously a clinical trial testing an experimental drug and an attempt to improve the lives of African women. But, as in similar trials, this mix proved difficult to negotiate. The vision and priorities of the MDP301 coordinators were not necessarily shared by trial participants. Following what it believed to be a strong code of ethics, the trial was nevertheless perceived by some to be exploitative and deadly. And despite promises of capacity building and safety, the specter of harmful trials continued to shape local perceptions of the MDP301. Most importantly, women's understandings of empowerment did not align with that of microbicide advocates. To grasp these complexities, we now turn to the MDP301's Johannesburg site and the township communities it impacted.

# Part 2

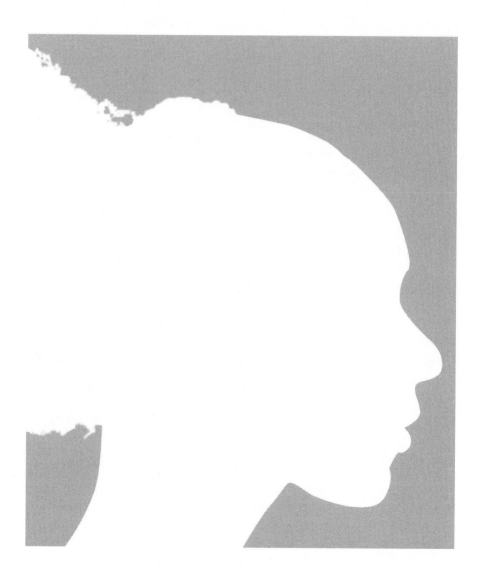

# Recruiting
# Meaning

The MDP301 prepared to begin its formal enrollment in 2005. Metropolitan Johannesburg, one of the South African sites for the trial, had a population of over four million, and coordinators were well aware that they would have to focus their efforts on circumscribed regions within the larger city. Wishing to recruit poor black women at risk of HIV, they selected two areas situated southwest of the center: Soweto and Orange Farm. While previous biomedical research had been conducted in these townships, the studies had been focused within clinic or hospital settings, involved few patients, and were often HIV treatment trials. As a result, the Johannesburg site of the MDP301 was regarded as "trial naïve." Needing to convince women who had never before participated in medical research to join the trial, the MDP301 employed long-standing advocacy narratives: if PRO 2000/5 was proven effective, it would potentially impact the health of hundreds of thousands of African women. Women should consider joining the trial to help others like them.

By the end of the trial in 2009, 3,828 women from Soweto and Orange Farm had been screened and 2,508 enrolled. Trial volunteers embodied the demographics of their communities: they were young, poor, and uneducated. The majority of women (51 percent) were between 18 and 24 years of age, while 18 percent was between 25 and 29, 13 percent was between 30 and 34, and 18 percent was over 35. Only 6 percent of participants had studied at the tertiary level, with the majority (89 percent) completing secondary school and 5 percent having finished only primary school. Most participants were unemployed (74 percent) and those with jobs accounted for only 13 percent of the study population.[1] To make ends meet, many participants relied on the financial assistance of a partner: 17 percent received all, 24 percent received half, and 20 percent received a third of household monies from a partner. The remaining women were the sole breadwinners in their households. While the MDP301 categorized its participants statistically, each woman was unique and had her own story and motivation for joining the trial.

Resigned to a life of "sitting at home," Mandisa was unemployed and, like many other women in Soweto, had all but given up on finding a secure job. Without a high school certificate it was impossible to get work, and even workers with certificates were restricted to cleaning jobs in government offices. This situation has worsened as the result of increasing competition from migrants from neighboring countries for menial jobs, and the negative attitudes of many employers toward Sowetans as "unreliable and lazy" (Ashforth 2005:27). Although Mandisa had worked as a waitress in a fast-food restaurant for several years, she was unemployed when she joined the trial and was relieved to find that the MDP301 would compensate her for taxi fare when visiting the clinic. Yet, she described herself as not really poor. Her sister supported the household, and Mandisa's lover, Siphiwe, a 38-year-old man from nearby Naledi, was employed at one of the major banks and had job stability. The couple first met in 2000 when Siphiwe was buying lunch at the restaurant where Mandisa worked. They became involved, but Mandisa was also seeing "a Zulu man" at the time, and she feared that he might become violent if he learned about Siphiwe, so she did not continue the new relationship. Four years later, Mandisa was visiting a friend and saw Siphiwe jogging. They swapped phone numbers and got back together. But they do not live together—not yet, not until they have a baby together. Although they both want a child, Mandisa will not entertain becoming pregnant until Siphiwe has an HIV test. Unlike Mandisa, who took the test regularly, he has never done so. To Mandisa, this may indicate that he knows that he is HIV positive and is too afraid to face facts. Hoping that the testing and counseling offered by the trial would help her resolve these issues, Mandisa joined the MDP301.

While residents like Mandisa saw the trial as potentially beneficial, others viewed it as a threat. For Thaba, the MDP301 seemed suspicious. He said bluntly, "I do not like white people's stuff because I am an African." Thaba was not alone. Despite the efforts made by the trial staff to disseminate a clear and positive message about the MDP301, rumors about the trial, its clinics, and personnel began appearing. Echoing accusations leveled in the press at other trials, community members spoke of the MDP301 as a front for malicious researchers intent on exposing Africans to HIV.[2] Although Mandisa's and Thaba's statements might appear to be quite different, both are born out of the context of South African townships. Situated within an environment of racial segregation, gender disparity, and economic hardship, the MDP301 came to embody a number of contrasting connotations. In seeking to recruit participants from the surrounding townships, the trial was transformed into a social actor imbued with meaning.

## SOWETO AND ORANGE FARM

Despite being geographically and historically distinct, Soweto and Orange Farm host some of the most impoverished neighborhoods in the country. Although an ever-increasing range of economic classes inhabits these communities, the area remains notorious for its pervasive poverty and violence. The highway spanning the thirty kilometers between the two townships is regarded as one of the most dangerous in the country. The population represents a wide range of ethnic identities, including Zulu, Sotho, Tswana, Venda, and Xhosa, and many households retain links to rural areas, as children and adults oscillate between their urban and rural homes (Gilbert and Crankshaw 1999; Saethre and Stadler 2009). But even as households are conscious of ethnicity, individuals more readily identify as urban dwellers, Sowetans, and Orange Farmers.

The South Western Townships, commonly known as Soweto, is a collective of 30 separate townships fused into a single urban conurbation. Soweto is the largest township in South Africa. Although the name Soweto was not adopted until 1963, the area's earliest black settlement—Kliptown—dates back to 1909, when it was laid out on former farmland (Bonner and Segal 1998). At the turn of the twentieth century, modern South Africa was born out of the devastation of the Anglo-Boer War. At the war's conclusion, the British colonies of the Cape and Natal were incorporated with the formerly independent South African Republic and the Orange Free State to form the Union of South Africa. Sitting atop the richest gold reef in the world, Johannesburg quickly became the economic center of the country. For the difficult work of gold extraction, the mines relied on black migrant laborers from around southern Africa. As the population of Johannesburg swelled with migrant laborers who now had sustained access to cash, the economic and social fabric of South Africa shifted. Currency replaced cattle as a means of prestige and exchange, while family relationships were restructured as men were separated from their wives, children, and land for extended periods (Murray 1981).

As rural Africans continued to seek work in Johannesburg, the need for more housing became acute, in part because of attempts to segregate the city center. In 1923, the Native Urban Areas Act was passed, preventing nonwhites from residing in urban areas. Until this time, the majority of Johannesburg's black working class had resided in "slum yards" within the city center. These spaces were "disease ridden" and considered to be unhealthy dens of interracial mixing (Bonner and Segal 1998). After a program of clearances and the demolition of the yards in the late 1920s and early 1930s, townships were created in an effort to keep pace with the rising number of migrants arriving in the city. Although yard residents were relocated to new townships and worker's hostels, others lacking the legal right to live in Johannesburg had to find alternatives as renters in the backyards of white homes or as squatters on the land surrounding the townships and mining hostels (ibid.; Crankshaw 2005).

After the Second World War, the Afrikaner-dominated National Party was elected and began a policy of apartheid. Determined to end the long history of mixed-race neighborhoods in Johannesburg, the government stepped up township construction in earnest. During the 1950s, small homes—labeled "matchboxes" because of their size—were built for Africans in what would come to be known as Soweto. As the years progressed, more and more townships were erected in the area. A distinctive feature of township development in the 1960s was the ethnic categorization of neighborhoods, a policy in line with Prime Minister Hendrik Verwoerd's ideology of separate development: "Those who belong together naturally want to live near one another, and the policy of ethnic grouping will lead to the development of an intensified community spirit" (quoted in Bonner and Segal 1998:9). Consequently, the townships of Naledi, Mapetla, Tladi, Moletsane, and Phiri were intended for Sotho and Tswana speakers, while Dhlamini, Senaoane, Zola, Zondi, Jabulani, Emdeni, and White City were built for Zulu and Xhosa speakers, and Tshiawelo was established for Tsonga and Venda speakers. This fragmentation was resisted by residents, who expressed a unified identity. Through strong community organizing and by speaking the local argot known as Tsotsitaal ("gangster language"), Sowetans resisted government attempts to shape their social world.

Throughout the 1970s and 1980s, economic upheavals paralleled social ones. In the 1970s, as gold prices boomed, the mines shifted to employing professional miners on longer-term contracts, but this period of relative stability was short lived. Increasing deindustrialization of the South African economy meant fewer and fewer investments in the mining sector, resulting in significant job losses. The number of skilled and even semi-skilled professions that once sustained the previous generations declined, and even the most menial jobs were fiercely fought over, pitting Soweto residents against migrants from neighboring states and rural areas (Ashforth 2005). As a poignant reminder of the decline of the mining industry, yellow mountains of sand stripped of gold dotted the city. Suffused with poverty, Soweto quickly became a major locus of the struggle against the apartheid regime. On 16 June 1976, during a march in which thousands of students protested against the imposition of the Afrikaans language as the medium of instruction in Soweto's schools, the police, who were untrained and unprepared, opened fire and killed several people in the crowd. Rioting followed and by the end of February 1977 the official death toll stood at 575 (Bonner and Segal 1998). The Soweto Uprising led to increasingly vocal opposition to apartheid around the world and transformed Soweto into the primary location through which educational and economic boycotts were organized. As a result of the role the township played in the struggle against apartheid, Sowetan identity remains a strong social marker.

When population controls were lifted after the end of apartheid in the early 1990s, the social separation of Soweto from Johannesburg disappeared, and in 2002, the township was formally incorporated into the city. Today, Soweto has approximately one million residents living in a diverse collection of homes: older township houses are juxtaposed between suburban mansions and sprawling squatter settlements. While South Africans are ever-mindful of its role in the struggle, Soweto has become a symbol of newfound black affluence. What has been described as the "boom period" of the early 2000s had a significant impact in urban areas such as Soweto, which has witnessed the growth of the black middle class and what is referred to in market research as the "super rich category of Black Elites" or "Black Diamonds" (Krige 2011:128). A centerpiece of the new Soweto, Maponya Mall, which cost R65 million ($6.5 million) and was opened by Nelson Mandela in 2007, is a place where the "trendy Sowetan community gather to shop, socialize, eat, and to see and be seen" (SOJO Business and Tourism Forum 2016).[3] Described as "a new monument to South African liberation" (Posel 2010), it is resplendent with brass elephants, water fountains, and a statue depicting Hector Pieterson, a victim of the 1976 revolt. Contributing to Soweto's already significant tourism market, similar developments are evident in the upgrading of old Kliptown, complete with a conference center and museum dedicated to the adoption of the 1955 Freedom Charter.[4] The growing affluence in some areas of Soweto embodies the new identities being adopted by young professional black elites, who have become more likely to leave Soweto and move to "white" suburbs.

In stark contrast to these signs of new wealth in parts of Soweto, the majority of the township's inhabitants remain poor urban "dust mongers" (Krige 2011). While comprehensive demographic data for Soweto is surprisingly absent, a University of the Witwatersrand survey conducted in the late 1990s documented extremely high rates of unemployment and poverty (Morris and Bozzoli 1999). Only 40 percent of the population over 16 years old was employed full time, and only a quarter of those between 20 and 29 years of age were employed at all (ibid., 8). Reflecting a rise in income disparity, levels of affluence were highly differentiated between households: a third earned less than R1,000 per month ($100), as part of the almost 60 percent earning less than R1,500 ($150) per month. Fifteen percent earned more than R3,000 ($300) per month, with only 5 percent of households enjoying an income greater than R5,000 ($500) per month (ibid., 10). These trends seem to have intensified in the mid- to late 2000s.

Although over the past two decades personal incomes and quality of life have improved for some Sowetans, many continue to depend on sources of welfare, such as pensions and child support grants (Ashforth 2005). In addition to contending with the challenges of living on a fixed income, they may endure the considerable social shame associated with being unable to support a family through wage labor and being over reliant on state welfare (MacGregor 2006). As overcrowding increases and housing costs rise, many Sowetans are renting space in backyards, building rudimentary shacks that lack adequate sanitation, water, and electricity. Goitsemedime is one of these individuals. She lives with her partner, Tau, in a shack at the back of a fenced Sowetan home. Goitsemedime left KwaZulu-Natal at the age of 18 to look for work in Soweto. Almost 30 years later, she jokes that although she didn't find a job, she did find a husband. Tau is a good man, she says, and he affectionately refers to her as Lovely. Together, they have raised two children who are now in their teens. Although Tau is working as a truck driver, Goitsemedime is still trying to find employment. As a result, they have been unable to afford a home of their own. The family of four lives in a small two-room shack, with one room serving as a kitchen and lounge area while the other acts as a bedroom. Goitsemedime and her family are not alone. An estimated 200,000 people are living in backyard houses in Soweto, accounting for almost one-fifth of the total Sowetan population and two-fifths of all households (Crankshaw et al. 2000).[5]

Goitsemedime's case not only illustrates the financial challenges confronting families, but also highlights the difficulties women face in accessing employment and, as a result, cash. Although unemployment is pervasive, men enjoy greater access to wage labor than do women. While it is socially acceptable for a woman such as Goitsemedime to be supported by a stable husband, young unmarried women are thought to gain their money illicitly, either through welfare payments or sex. It is believed that young women become pregnant on purpose just to receive the child support grant (Makiwane et al. 2006).[6] Their offspring are known as "Mbeki's children" because the former president championed the policy. While the popular media has portrayed women as incentivizing unprotected sex and teenage pregnancies, these claims have been refuted by researchers, who observe that access to welfare grants often means the difference between going hungry or not (Patel et al. 2012). But for many women, sexual transactions have indeed become a critical component of everyday survival (Hunter 2002; Jewkes et al. 2003; Kaufman and Stavrou 2002). In a survey of pregnant women in Soweto, 21 percent reported engaging in transactional sex, for which they received food (43 percent), clothing (36 percent), transport (30 percent), cosmetics (33 percent), items for children and families (13 percent), a place to sleep (11 percent), school fees (8 percent), and cash (94 percent) (Dunkle et al. 2004b). In Soweto, some women saw their boyfriends as "ATMs" or "checkbooks" (Wojcicki 2002a:360). In isiZulu, these transactions are called *ukuphanda*, which can be loosely translated as "try to get money," and are not associated with commercial sex work or prostitution (Hunter 2002; Wojcicki 2002a). Although these women were not referred to as prostitutes because they did not "stand in the streets," they were nevertheless accused of relentlessly pursuing money and, in the process, transforming love and relationships into commodities.[7]

While accessing cash through sex was viewed by many as illicit, it allowed women a degree of freedom and, for some, fun. Nomsa, for instance, reminisced about her late teen years, when she juggled five boyfriends. After a fight with the father of her first child, she moved to Soweto. Telling the men there that she was visiting the township only on specific days, Nomsa saw one on Monday, another on Tuesday, a third on Thursday or Friday, and the final two on weekends. Not only did they supply her with gifts, meals out, and cash, Nomsa enjoyed the thrill of deceiving them. She added that the father of her child never found out. Now Nomsa is in her twenties and in a stable relationship. Her partner doesn't talk a lot, but Nomsa said that she prefers quiet men. Her family has moved to Orange Farm, where Nomsa, her parents, and four siblings live in a three-room shack made of corrugated iron. She is happy with only one partner but intermittently yearns to take a secret lover. Having a variety of partners to choose from, she observed, was enjoyable. But Nomsa admits that she will never do this. Laughing, she remarked that she is no longer a teenager and doesn't have the energy for so much deception anymore.

However, unlike Nomsa, not all women enjoyed their relationships with men. For many, being reliant on a male left them vulnerable to coercion, mistreatment, and violence.[8] Although she was only 19 years old, Precious had struggled since becoming sexually mature. As was typical, her household was supported by a male, her father. When Precious entered puberty, her father began to suspect that she was engaging in illicit sex with neighborhood boys. As punishment, he locked Precious in her room and beat her. Assuming that she was being supported by these presumed lovers, her father stopped giving Precious money and would not let her eat any of the food in the home. Without a source of support, Precious moved into a shelter. However, after only a few months, the owner's son raped Precious. Precious told the owner what had occurred but her story was not believed. The owner said Precious had been the aggressor, seducing her son in hopes of getting money from him. Precious was summarily evicted from the shelter. With no place else to go, she alternated between staying with friends and living on the street. After a few weeks, Precious met Thaba. He wanted to take things slowly but because she was homeless, he invited her to move in with him. Although she is now dependent on Thaba for support, Precious is unsure about their relationship. Like her father, Thaba has begun accusing her of seeing other men. Meanwhile, she suspects that he might be having an affair with the mother of his child. With no money and no familial support, Precious has little choice but to continue staying with Thaba.

Given the economic difficulties facing many people in Soweto, families such as Nomsa's have moved away in an attempt to establish their own households. A popular choice of destination is Orange Farm. Orange Farm acquired its name from the color of its soil, where white landowners had previously grown a variety of vegetable and cereal crops, as well as prospecting for diamonds (Crankshaw 1993). Similar to Soweto's, Orange Farm's beginnings as a township can be traced to population removals and the resettlement of urban inhabitants, albeit in a different era. In the mid-1980s, steady decline in industrial development on the West Rand resulted in massive job losses and the growth of a homeless and jobless underclass. Soweto was already overcrowded, and as blacks sought housing, farm-lands were transformed into townships in the peri-urban areas of western Johannesburg, rendering former farm workers landless. Seeing an opportunity, the registered white owners of Orange Farm, the Weiler brothers, allowed families to erect shacks and use existing supplies of potable water in exchange for a small monthly rent. Although much of the surrounding area was expropriated for township development, Orange Farm remained private land until 1987. However, after the death of one of the Weiler brothers, the farm was flooded by settlers: in two years, from 1985 to 1987, the number of families increased from 70 to 1,110 (Crankshaw and Hart 1990). Many of the initial residents were homeless people from the numerous townships surrounding the industrial towns of Vereeniging and Vanderbijlpark, as well as backyard shack dwellers from Soweto.[9] As the years progressed, continued overcrowding in Soweto ensured that Orange Farm received a steady stream of migrants seeking available land.

Because Orange Farm is roughly equidistant from surrounding urban areas, no local authority was willing to take responsibility for the welfare of its inhabitants. This neglect, combined with its remoteness, meant that its residents were left alone to build their homes in a "no–man's–land" without the constant harassment experienced by "squatters" in similar "squatter camps" established in or closer to Johannesburg. Unlike the residents of other townships, Orange Farmers were allowed to control their own homes without interference from landlords. A shack in Orange Farm offered privacy and freedom one could not find elsewhere. Land could be purchased for R500 ($50) or rented for R20 ($2) per month, allowing dispossessed people permanency. As a result of the lack of regulation and standardization, Orange Farm's streets and houses have a very different look from those of Soweto. Dwellings are unlike the thousands of replica matchbox houses constructed by the 1950s Nationalist Party government or, indeed, the "RDP" two-room structures built by the ANC-led government more recently. It is not unusual to see rudimentary shacks standing next to mini-mansions with high walls and elaborately designed wrought-iron gates.

Over the years, Orange Farm has continued to represent the hope of owning land and a better future for the poor, which has created a strong sense of common identity within the area as a whole. Chris Hani, the leader of the South African Communist Party from 1991 until his assassination in 1993, renamed the township "Palestine" in recognition of the parallels between the struggle of black South Africans for land and those of the Palestinian people (Stadler et al. 2013). Throughout the 1990s, Orange Farm was a choice destination for international donors. The numerous schools, early childhood development centers, and Internet centers are testimonies to these investments, as is a community center that boasts an Olympic-size swimming pool and a gym. Since the first free elections in 1994, Orange Farm, like Soweto, has seen increasing development dovetail with the building of monuments celebrating the struggle against apartheid: in 1999 the Chris Hani-Nike Sports Stadium was opened.

But, as in Soweto, the construction of new facilities has done little to improve the everyday lives of most Orange Farmers. Orange Farm remains one of the poorest areas in greater Johannesburg. Statistics regarding income, education, illness, and housing repeatedly demonstrate the challenges facing its residents. Compared to other areas of Johannesburg, the community has the highest proportion of people without any education (8 percent) and people who are "too sick to work" (16 percent) (De Wet et al. 2008). Orange Farmers frequently have difficulty feeding themselves and their families, with only 10 percent reporting food security (ibid.). Because of the large number of female-headed households, there is also a higher prevalence of parents accessing the child support grant. A lack of central planning has resulted in few people having access to potable water inside their homes, with most relying on external taps and pit latrines. When water meters were installed on these taps in some sections of Orange Farm, households quickly ran out of water early in the month, having used up their allocated six kiloliters of water per household per month of "free water." The Orange Farm Water Crisis Committee was formed and frequently leads protests. In 2006, blockades of the Golden Highway were staged, with protesters demanding decent water, electricity, and sanitation.

Like many township dwellers, the Orange Farmers we interviewed were acutely aware that they lacked the services and wealth that other South

Africans enjoyed. Thaba, for instance, often remarked on South Africa's pervasive inequality. Raised in a former homeland, Thaba's father left him when he was young. His mother moved the rest of the family to Soweto, seeking economic opportunities, but she was unable to make ends meet and took him from one home to another. Participating in the mass protests in Soweto during apartheid, Thaba wanted to change South Africa for the better. After leaving home, he moved to Orange Farm to start his own family. However, this has not happened as he had hoped. Although two of his previous girlfriends became pregnant, they each miscarried. Looking back, Thaba suspects that the women actually lied to him and underwent abortions because he was unemployed and politically active. Young men like Thaba often cannot afford to establish and support a family. In addition to finding housing, men must also pay *lobola* or bridewealth. Over the years, the price of *lobola* has risen alongside the cash economy, leading an increasing number of men to complain that taking a wife and starting a family have become ever more costly and prohibitive (Kaler 2006).

Unable to pay *lobola*, Thaba could not convince his earlier partners that their relationships would be stable. He did eventually find a girlfriend who became pregnant and gave birth to a baby girl. Thaba's initial joy at becoming a father was quickly transformed into anxiety. Suspecting that the child's mother was having affairs, he worried about whether she would infect his daughter with HIV via her breastmilk. After publicly accusing his partner of being an unfit parent, he sent the baby to live with his family. Although Thaba is now in a new relationship with Precious, who adores his daughter, he cannot be reunited with his child. Without a steady income, Thaba cannot raise her himself. Now 34 years old, Thaba is angry because she is enduring the same circumstances that he did as a child. He had dreamed of passing what he proudly called his African values to his many children, but without a job, he conceded, that would not happen.

## ENROLLING PARTICIPANTS

The MDP301 chose Soweto and Orange Farm in large part because of the high rates of poverty, unemployment, violence, and HIV. But trial coordinators also acknowledged that these factors would impact enrollment as concerns abounded regarding the site's ability to recruit three thousand participants. Assuming that a significant number of women would be ineligible after their initial screening, the MDP301 estimated that approximately six thousand women would have to be seen before the target was reached. Unlike HIV and cancer treatment trials, the MDP301 required volunteers who were at risk of HIV and who were prepared to use an experimental product. While treatment trials often attracted a large number of willing volunteers seeking medication, the MDP301 would have to convince healthy women to join. The ways in which trial coordinators designed and implemented the recruitment, screening, and enrollment process reflected their goals of the MDP301 being statistically sound, ethical, and positively impactful. But for women such as Mandisa, the actual experience of enrollment was fraught with uncertainty and apprehension.

Anticipating that recruitment could be difficult, the MDP301 began an intensive campaign a year prior to the official launch of the trial. Although overall management of the MDP301 trial was through the Medical Research Council Clinical Trials Unit and Imperial College London, the clinics and recruitment efforts in Soweto and Orange Farm were coordinated locally by Wits Reproductive Health and HIV Institute (then known as the Reproductive Health Research Unit or RHRU). While government clinics were regarded as the optimal enrollment settings, their staff initially resisted microbicide research. Fearing that the MDP301 would harm participants and encourage them to have more sex, public health officials denied trial staff access to clinics. HIV counselors at one clinic in Soweto confronted MDP301 community health workers, saying that PRO 2000/5 caused AIDS. The counselors were aware of the closure of the CS trial and referenced a newspaper article posted on the clinic wall that asserted microbicides were harmful. Although MDP301 coordinators considered Soweto and Orange Farm trial naïve, community members had already been exposed to media stories about microbicides and their trials. After trial staff addressed these reports and provided extensive consultation, permission was eventually granted and recruitment activities began in these clinics.

Having won over clinic staff, trial coordinators shifted their message to potential volunteers, who often expressed misgivings about joining. On one occasion, two community health workers met with patients at an Orange Farm clinic, speaking about the previous studies undertaken by RHRU and the search for methods that would work in addition to condoms to prevent HIV. Nine men and twenty-eight women listened to the presentation and asked a number of questions, including why condom use was promoted by the trial when condoms had been shown to be unsafe, how the trial would know if the gel was effective if women were using it with condoms as instructed, and what researchers would do if people tested positive for HIV either during their initial screening or later, after they had been enrolled. On this occasion, the community health workers found these questions difficult to answer.[10] The male patients were particularly vocal, challenging the community health workers to alleviate their concerns about the trial exposing women to HIV and putting their own lives at risk. These questions and issues would be raised repeatedly by potential volunteers, participants, and their partners throughout the duration of the trial. At the end of the presentation, nine of the women present said that they were interested in the study, while nineteen were not.

As the start date for the trial approached, the staff of the MDP301 turned their attention to recruiting volunteers in public, on the roadside, in shopping malls, and during health awareness days. Community health workers set up stalls and handed out pamphlets about microbicides. Individuals displaying an interest in the trial were asked to come to the clinic for screening. In addition, a media campaign focused attention on the MDP301 through community radio. A number of radio shows routinely discussed the importance of HIV prevention, and the trial used these platforms to advertise and seek recruits. A show branded *Tshireletso Health Talk* was particularly popular and seemed to stimulate women's interest as well as to legitimize the MDP301 by providing clear information about the trial (Medeossi et al. 2014). While radio was an effective recruitment tool, word of mouth proved to be the main reason women came to the trial clinics for screening. Like many participants, Mandisa obtained information about the MDP301 from more than one source before deciding to be screened: "I heard about it on the radio and I kept telling myself that I would go. I wanted to join. My little sister at home is a nurse, and when I told her about what I heard, she told me to just go and join the study. She told me that it was going to help me but I never got around to doing it. Eventually, my little cousin's sister came and she told me more about that study and also told me that I should join. Then eventually I went to the clinic and I ended up enrolling." Later, Mandisa added, "I wanted to do blood tests, Pap smears, and I wanted to know my health in general, if I was still fine." Many women echoed Mandisa's statement, saying that they too had enrolled to learn more about their health. Precious commented, "It was just knowing or being updated about my health status that I appreciated." Although trial recruitment messages stressed the importance of finding an alternative to condoms, enrollment was predominantly motivated by the regular medical testing and care offered by the MDP301.

Once women made the decision to be screened, they were required to attend one of the two trial clinics. The Soweto clinic was located within the security fences of Chris Hani Baragwanath Hospital, one of the largest in the world. Participants needed to wind their way around hospital buildings amid the congestion of patients and staff to get to the clinic. The waiting area featured a long but relatively narrow hallway lined with chairs on the one side and doors to consultation rooms on the other. Television sets were mounted up on the walls for participants to watch as they waited their turn. In contrast to the tumult of Chris Hani Baragwanath Hospital, the Orange Farm clinic was located on a dirt track not far off the main road through the township. Situated in a neighborhood of tiny two-bedroomed cinder block and tin houses, the clinic space was small. On busy days, participants squeezed in next to each other, sharing space on the plastic chairs, craning their necks to watch the kung fu and Nigerian horror movies screened on the television. Staff space was similarly intimate; the physician of record shared his office with filing cabinets. Yet, the physical intimacy and hectic pace of the clinic created an almost festive atmosphere: women waiting for their appointments would sooner or later begin chatting about sex, relationships, and their experiences of using the gel. In both clinics the amount of time spent waiting to see a clinician could be extreme. It was not uncommon for women to arrive in the morning and not leave until the afternoon. Several participants complained about the long waits wasting their time, noting that they had active lives and needed the time for running errands, job hunting, and caring for household members.

Women experienced a range of emotions and anxieties throughout every step of the screening and enrollment process. Like many others, Mandisa was extremely nervous about coming into the clinic for the first time because she knew that she would be screened for HIV. She said, "I felt bad because I was afraid to do the HIV test. I mean many people are afraid to do HIV tests and it is normal." After clinic staff went over the screening procedures and informed consent, Mandisa, like other potential participants, was counseled about her potential risk for HIV infection. She revealed that her partner was dishonest and that she had occasionally cared for an ill relative, and feared having contracted HIV accidently: "I was somewhat afraid when they were taking blood. Even though I knew I was playing safe I had some fears because

I did not trust my partner. And sometimes you find that one of the siblings is not feeling well and you have to help him and accidents may happen and you get an infection." Mandisa was so nervous that she even considered walking out: "I thought of stopping but I stood bold and continued to do the tests." Her response was common for many volunteers: they wanted to be tested for HIV but were nonetheless extremely worried about the results. Like all potential participants, Mandisa was given a rapid test, which was performed on a dried blood spot, but nurses also drew venous blood for a confirmatory ELISA (enzyme-linked immunosorbent assay) test. Mandisa was pleased to learn that she was HIV negative and eligible to continue the screening process. However, her results did not dispel her fears, as the nurses had informed her about the window period during which seroconversion could occur. While initially testing HIV negative was likewise a relief for many other women, they too remained uncertain and anxious about their status. Andiswa commented, "It's scary! Even though I know that I am HIV negative, it is still scary because I know there is a window period and in three months' time, the results could come back different. It is scary to take any blood test." It was only through repeated and regular testing during the trial that these women would come to feel more secure about their health.

Potential participants who tested HIV negative and were not pregnant, like Mandisa, were invited back for a second enrollment screening. During this visit, further counseling sessions were held, genital examinations were performed, additional blood samples were taken, and trial staff reviewed a comprehension checklist with potential participants to ensure that key trial guidelines were understood. While women coming back for their second appointment did not have the stress associated with undergoing an HIV test, many were apprehensive about the genital exam. For some, this was their first experience of this kind of procedure. The clinician used a speculum, and a swab was taken only if vaginal discharge was observed. There were very few physical complaints regarding the exam—a cold speculum and some subsequent slight menstrual spotting were the most frequently mentioned issues—but many women found the procedure to be uncomfortable socially. Women felt embarrassed exposing their bodies to medical staff, particularly male doctors. To alleviate their concerns, a female nurse was instructed to be present at these exams. However, younger women were also uneasy when an older female clinician conducted the inspection, as it revealed that they were sexually active. One participant reported, "I was worried because the woman who did it was much older than I am. I was worried about what she was going to think of me. She might have seen me as somebody who is loose or without any moral standards. But I got used to it." Several women who were nervous prior to the examination were put at ease as they spoke to the clinicians and established rapport. A participant recalled,

> I do not like it when someone looks at me here [pointing to her groin] and I also do not like it when my partner looks at my vagina. So, that is why I do not expect a complete stranger to look at it. But the person who examined me was very good. She asked me to lie down and she comforted me that it will be fine. And we started chatting and I did not realize that she was examining me at that time. And suddenly she told me that she has finished and I was surprised because I did not feel anything. She was very good and she communicated with me in a friendly manner and she made me feel at ease. They treat people well.

While most of the women were nervous about the genital exam, their responses to the event itself were varied, and overall their experiences were positive.

Although many participants spoke of experiencing social discomfort during their exams, most felt this was far outweighed either by the benefits of early disease detection and treatment or by the relief of being given a clean bill of health: "I am happy to be in a study where they conduct all these examinations because I would have never known about my infection or I would have found out about it when it was a bit too late for them to treat it. Being a part of this study has helped me a lot." A significant proportion of trial participants were diagnosed and treated for sexually transmitted infections and other genital ailments. According to the clinical data collected, 46.5 percent (1144/2298) of women who were enrolled had the genital herpes simplex virus (HSV-2), 3 percent (77) had syphilis, 8.1 percent (202) tested positive for trichomonas vaginalis, 3 percent (74) for gonorrhea, and 12 percent (310) for chlamydia. In some cases problems more serious than infections were discovered. During one enrollment examination, a participant was diagnosed with a prolapsed uterus and referred to gynecological services at Chris Hani Baragwanath Hospital. She said, "I did not know about it. The only thing I felt was that whenever I was sneezing or laughing I had pain in my genitals. Sometimes I felt the pain even when I was sitting down, but I did not know what the problem was." Like many other women, she had not sought treatment for these symptoms prior to joining the trial. Involvement in the MDP301 was therefore a means not only of accessing regular HIV testing but also of ensuring reproductive health.

While women spoke of HIV testing and genital exams as stressful but necessary, this was not the case for blood draws, another regular component of trial participation. During a woman's second visit, 20 milliliters (ml) of blood (four tubes) were taken to test for HSV-2 and syphilis as well as to store for future tests. In addition, the first 500 women enrolled in the trial gave 15 ml of blood for full blood counts to assess liver and kidney function and for clotting tests. Venous blood draws also occurred on follow-up visits and were taken at least five times throughout the duration of a participant's enrollment in the trial. The rationale for regular testing was well understood by trial participants, but the blood draws, especially the volume of blood taken at certain visits, caused anxiety: "They are taking too much blood! For instance, last time I came here they took about seven or eight tubes. I told the nurse that I am afraid when they take blood." When women expressed their apprehension, clinic staff did not always provide adequate responses:

> I asked them, "Why are you taking so much blood?" and they said that they had to take it and then I just kept quiet and let them take it. . . . They told me that they were taking the blood to do the test in the laboratory. Then I asked them why they were not using one bottle [test tube] of blood and then they told me that one bottle would be taken to this and that place. They used their medical terms that I could not understand.

To address such perceptions, clinic staff counseled participants and showed them how little blood was actually drawn—that twenty ml of blood only equaled four teaspoons.

Participants' physical experiences added to the perception that excessive blood was being taken: "After they have taken blood you feel uncomfortable, weak, and dizzy." Participants and nonparticipants alike widely viewed the blood draws as debilitating, leading some family members to voice concern: "My grandmother was complaining that I have lost too much weight because of the blood that I keep on losing all the time I come to the clinic. Then my aunt said she won't come and participate because of the blood that we always lose." The issue of blood draws caused some women to hesitate before volunteering for the trial. After enrolling, one woman said, "Even myself, I did not agree to come here the first time I heard about the clinic. It took me a while to come. . . . I had heard that they take a lot of blood. I did not know about the gels but I knew about drawing of blood." Although HIV tests and physical exams were thought to facilitate better health through accurate diagnosis, blood draws were thought to imperil health.

The final step prior to enrollment was confirming that potential participants clearly understood three key points. Clinicians completed a comprehension checklist for every potential participant. The MDP301 strove to make sure that women knew they were using either an experimental product or a placebo; they were not to use the gel as their sole HIV prevention method. Consequently, the first statement on the checklist was "The gel may not protect her from HIV." The checklist suggested asking the participant, "How certain are you that the gel you receive in this trial will protect you against HIV or other STIs?" The clinician was to proceed only if the answer indicated uncertainty. Again concerned that the gel would be used in isolation, the second checklist item was "Condoms will protect her from HIV." Throughout the trial, all participants were told to use condoms in tandem with the gel. Clinicians were advised to ask, "What sort of things can you do to prevent yourself getting infected with HIV?" and needed to hear the word "condom" in reply. The final statement was "She will have to stop using the gel if she becomes pregnant." Clinicians were urged to verify women's agreement to this stipulation—that each participant knew she would have to cease using the gel permanently and drop out of the trial if she conceived a child.

In addition to these three key points, another three were also listed as "important":

1. She understands that she can withdraw from the study at any time. [On clinicians' copies of the checklist, this point was underlined.]
2. She knows that MRC is the sponsor of the trial.
3. She knows who to contact in case of any problem relating to the gel.

The comprehension checklist was yet another tool to ensure that potential participants accepted specific trial messages prior to enrollment. Throughout their participation, women would be repeatedly reminded of these dominant messages and asked to demonstrate their understanding of them. Once the comprehension checklist was completed, women were officially enrolled

## GEL INSTRUCTIONS

1. Make sure you have dry hands. Remove the prefilled applicator and plunger from the sealed wrapper.

2. Place the small end of the plunger into the hole at the back end of the applicator (the end opposite the blue cap).

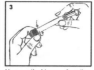

3. Unscrew the blue cap from the smooth end of the applicator. Throw the blue cap away.

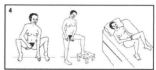

4. Choose a comfortable position, for example, squatting with your feet apart, standing with one leg raised, or lying on your back with your knees apart.

5. Measure 3-4 fingers from the top of the applicator. (not including the plunger)

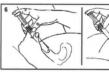

6. Glently insert the applicator into your vagina until your fingers touch your body. Be careful not to insert the applicator too far. While holding the applicator firmly in place, push the plunger until it stops. Alternatively, you can hold the applicator steady with one hand, and then push the plunger down with the other.

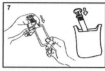

7. Withdraw the applicator from the vagina and put the used applicator and plunger back into the bag or wrapper so that you can return them to the clinic at your next visit.

IDEALLY YOU SHOULD APPLY THE GEL JUST BEFORE INTERCOURSE.

If intercourse does not occur within 1 hour of the gel being inserted, another applicator should be used to apply more gel in order to try to ensure that gel is used within an hour of intercourse.

**FIGURE 3.** Instructions on applying the gel. Courtesy of the Microbicide Development Program.

and randomized, and then sent to the pharmacy to collect their first month's supply of gel.

After successfully finishing all of the enrollment steps, participants were given R150 ($15). Per guidelines set by the Medicines Control Council of South Africa, trial participants across the country were reimbursed the same amount for every clinic visit. Over the course of the twelve-month enrollment period, participants came to the clinic for an appointment at least once a month. Women thus would receive a total sum of R1,800 ($180) for clinical appointments alone. In addition, those taking part in the social science in-depth interviews or making additional trips to the clinic received R50 ($5) for each visit, also per Medicines Control Council guidelines. Wanting to stress that women were volunteers and not paid for their participation, trial staff repeatedly asserted that this money was to reimburse travel expenses. However, the actual travel cost per appointment was far lower than R150, leading some to question the veracity of the clinic's assertions.

While the trial attempted to disseminate accurate and standardized information, these messages were not always understood or interpreted in the way that the MDP301 intended. When women posed questions, trial staff sometimes lacked the knowledge or time to answer them satisfactorily. If staff or nurses did not explain procedures adequately, women sought other sources. In trying to make sense of the MDP301 protocols, participants were influenced by friends, partners, and family members, who often had not been exposed to trial messages. In addition, women's experiences of the screening and trial process affected their perceptions of the trial just as much, if not more, than the MDP301 messages. For instance, the use of a speculum and swabs during the genital screenings led many participants, such as Mandisa, to believe that they were receiving Pap smears and being assessed for cervical cancer or abnormal cell growth. In fact, this was not the case. Similarly, although nurses attempted to demonstrate that the amount of blood being drawn was minimal, women felt their blood loss was excessive. When the trial produced unconvincing answers that seemed to contradict women's experiences, participants drew their own conclusions about the MDP301's goals and procedures.

## THE DANGER OF HIV PREVENTION INITIATIVES

As increasing numbers of women visited the trial clinics and enrolled, Sowetans and Orange Farmers began to take notice. Why, they asked, was an HIV prevention trial being conducted in their township? In stark contrast to microbicide advocates' narratives of hope and empowerment or participants' desire to monitor their health and HIV status, residents cast the MDP301 as a fundamentally harmful endeavor. Soon after recruitment efforts began and the first participants enrolled, a number of stories began circulating that asserted that the gels contained deadly substances—most commonly HIV. Community members, clinic staff, trial participants, and the clinical trial's community advisory group all reported hearing rumors that the MDP301 was designed to take the lives of unsuspecting Africans. While most participants discounted these stories, they were nevertheless acutely aware of them. Not confined to the MDP301, these rumors echoed a widespread trend in sub-Saharan Africa in which medical practice and research are a source of popular stories about blood theft (Geissler 2005a), the manufacture and spread of deadly diseases such as HIV (Niehaus and Jonsson 2005; Pool et al. 2001; Stadler 2003), sterility related to health products (Kaler 2009), and the trade in or theft of body parts (Campion-Vincent 2002; Scheper-Hughes 1996).

Marshaling social, economic, medical, and historical evidence, South Africans have consistently constructed local explanations of health crises. In the 1990s when the HIV/AIDS epidemic exploded in South Africa, the country was transitioning from apartheid to majority rule. Whereas HIV/AIDS in the United States seemed to affect gay men disproportionately, in South Africa it was black heterosexuals who bore the brunt of the epidemic. As township residents watched their family and friends succumb to the disease, they did not see white people sharing their experience. One man asked, "Do you remember the time we had the first vote and white people were not dying? Very few white people had AIDS." The history of racial inequality, coupled with the timing of the onset of the epidemic in South Africa, led many to postulate a connection between the two. The man, like many others, concluded that HIV/AIDS "is something that came from white people." Throughout Orange Farm and Soweto, HIV was regularly regarded as a disease created by white people for the express purpose of genocide. Some blamed Wouter Basson, a cardiologist and former head of "Project Coast," South Africa's biological warfare project, during the apartheid era, while others implicated American organizations such as the CIA.

Not only were whites blamed for the creation of the disease, but HIV prevention technologies such as condoms were seen as ways through which the virus was purposely spread. A participant speaking about the views of her neighbors commented, "Most people think things like condoms that are made by white people are the things that give black people diseases." To prove the veracity of these rumors, some individuals conducted informal experiments, such as placing an unrolled condom in a cup of hot water. Witnesses remarked that a greasy film quickly formed on the surface of the water. While some viewed the film as either lubricant or spermicidal gel, it indicated to others the presence of viral worms containing HIV. These observations were often bolstered by personal experiences of disease and death. For instance, despite the hot water test, Godson had remained skeptical about claims that condoms contained HIV, but he changed his opinion once a close family member died of AIDS. However, Godson was careful to note that only Choice brand condoms—those distributed free by the government and the MDP301—were infected with HIV. White people, he said, knew that untainted condoms could be found for sale in stores. Safe condoms were those that were purchased—a category out of reach for many poor black South Africans.

Given that HIV infection was linked to race, inequality, and prevention technologies, it was not surprising that the MDP301 was incorporated into these narratives. Participants and community members were acutely aware that the trial was primarily administered by whites. A participant noted, "People are asking why do they have names of white people in the pamphlets and why do they want to do research on black people and not on white people." The answer for some Sowetans and Orange Farmers was genocide. One man commented that if his partner had not spoken to him honestly about her participation in the trial, he would have been suspicious: "On many things, especially a project that was run by white people in a black township, I would have told myself that they are trying to finish us off." Narratives of malicious whites often portrayed the gel, like condoms, as a tool to bring about the death of Africans through deliberate HIV infection. These claims were seemingly supported by media reports of other microbicide clinical trials that had been discontinued or altered as a result of concerns about increased risk of HIV infection. The South African media coverage of the discontinuation of the CS trial particularly impacted views of the MDP301. Limpho reported, "My partner is supportive but since yesterday—after hearing that there were people who were using the gel and they became HIV positive—he started to panic, saying, 'You see that gel of yours!' He does not trust it [the gel] anymore."

While some residents marshaled media reports as evidence of the harmfulness of the trial, others highlighted the cash reimbursements received by participants. Women repeatedly remarked that the R50–R150 ($5-$15) they were given far exceeded the cost of transport, leading many to speculate about the "real" purpose of these payments. In some instances, the reimbursement was said to be a "bribe" intended to discourage participants from complaining about any side effects that resulted from gel use. In others, payments were cast as the primary method through which women were lured to their deaths. A male resident of Soweto recounted:

> The people who stay next to me are scared because someone came here [to the MDP301 clinic]. I mean at the time the research had just started and when they tested her they found that she is HIV positive. Then after three days she started to become very sick and then after that she died. So, people are scared because they said when you come here they tell you your status, then give you R50, and the next day after drinking a cold drink that you bought with the money that they give you, you die. They say it's better to stay without knowing your status.

Reimbursements, and the commodities purchased with the cash, were enticing but dangerous. Residents equated accepting money from the trial with "buying your coffin." As one woman succinctly stated, "They say you will die for the sake of getting R150."

Reimbursements were also the focus of another persistent narrative: according to residents, the trial exploited and harmed women by paying them a pittance for the blood that was drawn. This rumor was so well known that community members referred to the trial clinic as "money for blood" (isiZulu: *imali ye gazi*). While R150 was far more than the cost of transport, it was considered meager compensation for an individual's blood, which was viewed as an inherently valuable resource. Consequently, cash reimbursements were often referred to as "little money," particularly in regards to the amount of blood perceived to be collected. Community members accused the trial of deriving profit from reselling participant blood at high prices. As women were being cheated and kept in poverty, trial coordinators became wealthy: "They [community members] will say the clinic staff gets a lot of money from their blood because they even drive fancy cars and they give us a little money." Indeed, the observation that clinic staff drove "fancy cars" was true to a certain extent; the parking areas around both clinics contained an array of late-model vehicles. However, not only were women being exploited for cash, but their lives were put at risk. A participant revealed, "They [community members] normally say . . . we are going to die because we will end up being the ones who do not have enough blood." Blood was described as finite, rather than as a renewable resource. Consequently, excessive blood draws could debilitate the body, leading to sickness and death.

As these narratives circulated around the community, many participants dismissed tales of HIV-contaminated gels and blood selling as false. Despite news coverage of the CS trial and the concerns of her partner, Limpho did not believe that the MDP301 was endangering her health. She commented, "You know when we talk like this we must know that the media lies sometimes or exaggerates things; they add inaccurate information to get people's attention." Another participant claimed that these accusations were part of a larger pattern of suspicion occurring throughout South Africa. She said, "Everything that is new and is going to protect people from HIV, they say that is the thing that is going to cause HIV." Popular statements critiquing the trial elicited rebukes from participants, who often did not view the trial as dangerous or themselves as greedy. In a focus group, one participant recalled, "We were very angry about the media coverage that we were being used as these guinea pigs, that we had been bought by money to take part in the trial, and that we were selling our blood for money. They said black people are so poor we can be bought to join a clinical trial. But I am not so poor that I can sell myself for the R150 we got for transport." Women often stressed their dignity and agency, asserting that they certainly had not been lured or duped into participation.

While most participants rejected narratives of white malice, this was not universal. A few participants worried that perhaps the rumors were accurate, while others were apprehensive about side effects that could be caused by gel use. We were told that some women who did not "trust" the gel "dumped" it, emptying the applicator's contents into a toilet or sink. Consequently, narratives that accused the gel of being a harmful product impacted not only enrollment but also gel use. Although none of the women we interviewed admitted to dumping the gel, many claimed either to know or to have heard about gel dumpers. A few women attributed gel dumping to fear of using an experimental product: "For some it was fear because it is research. What if something goes wrong? Why are they testing it on us?" Others credited rumors of harm: "I think they are not using the gel because they hear those ones saying things like the gel has HIV and asking why do they give you money, so why is the money for free." Given stories of gels laced with HIV, gel dumping could be seen as a way for women to exercise their agency against a deadly trial. However, community residents did not applaud the actions of dumpers, but rather cast them as immoral.

Depicting participants as greedy, deceitful, and licentious, community residents expressed little sympathy for their plight, simultaneously regarding them as victims and moral weaklings. According to the rumors of coffin money and blood selling, the real reason that women joined the trial—risking their health and their lives in the process—was a selfish desire for "money all the time." Women who "sold their blood" did so because they "loved money" and "think they deserve to be paid for their blood." Participants were lazy, self-centered, and untrustworthy—accessing cash without participating in the wage labor market. A community member commented, "They [trial participants] did not work for that money. It is free and it is easy money." In addition, these greedy women concealed their gel use and reimbursements from their partners.[11] Lesedi observed, "You find that some women don't tell their partners that they are using the gel and they get 150 from the research that they are doing here. When she gets home she pretends as if she is not getting anything." One individual compared trial participants to the women who took advantage of government child support grants: "The money that they give people here in the clinic is like Thabo Mbeki's money [child grants] because you find that their boyfriends support their children but they still want the money from grants." Young women were particularly criticized for engaging in this behavior. A woman in her twenties said, "If you can say there is no longer money for attending the clinic you will see a miracle: only older people will remain in this clinic." A male Orange Farmer echoed these remarks, stating, "The older people don't do things like that because they are mature, so youngsters tell each other to go and join the trial so they can get money." Many also suggested that the greedy women accessing the trial for cash were engaging in sexual relations with numerous men, and some likened participants to prostitutes.

Dishonest women were regularly implicated in stories of gel dumping: "A person will go into the [bath]room for hours, squeezing the gel out so that they hand over an empty applicator. They are not using the gel. They are only coming here for money." During one community discussion, the following conversation took place:

*Woman 1*: They are not using it; they throw it away, you know, there where there is long grass they throw it there. When you go there you can see it and when they are finished squirting out the gel they put it in the plastic bag, then close it. Then they lie and say they used it. Meanwhile, they did not.

*Woman 2*: I saw other people using the gel. So if there are people who throw the gel away, it is those naughty ones you see.

*Woman 3*: I think they want money—the R150.

*Woman 2*: They are supposed to give the gel to people who are partners. Then they should tell them that they are giving them this gel because your [HIV] status is like this, and then they should agree with them that they are going to use the gel and that it is not just people who are there to play.

This exchange sums up many of the beliefs regarding gel dumpers: they are young, promiscuous, and deceitful. Like other greedy participants, gel dumpers spend their cash selfishly, purchasing jeans, getting their hair done, and buying Kentucky Fried Chicken. They also conceal their participation from partners: "It is just being naughty, because the majority of people dumping the gel are young people and those who did not disclose to their partners and they are only interested in money." Remarkably, other narratives accused women of deceiving their partners in an opposite fashion: by revealing their participation in the trial but not their dumping activities. In one case, a participant described a woman who pretended to insert the gel in front of her partner as a means of concealing her dishonesty. But gel dumpers were also misleading the trial by claiming that they had used the gel. When discussing her opinions about gel dumpers, one woman said, "It is not right because they are just playing with RHRU [the trial coordinator]."

Although they as a group were portrayed negatively, trial participants tended to support many of these popular narratives. They asserted that many women on the trial had indeed enrolled solely for the money, lied to their partners, and dumped the gel. Like others, Kagiso believed younger participants were highly likely to dump the gel. As proof, she recalled a conversation between "young girls" in the waiting room: "They said they would not use the gel because their boyfriends do not like it. I ended up asking them if they know this gel really works. Then they stopped talking." Kagiso, like every participant with whom we spoke, was careful to note that unlike others, she was not motivated by greed. Adopting an explicitly moralizing discourse, Zinzi commented, "Would people come without money? No, because most people who have joined the study are youngsters. They wouldn't come if there was no money. I heard about the study from one woman who stays in Soweto. I couldn't join then because I didn't have money for transport. But I was doing an HIV test at Sebokeng Hospital, although I didn't do the genital examination. I told you that money doesn't mean a lot. What matters most is my life." Zinzi, who was 41 years old at the time, emphasized that unlike these young women, she was in a stable relationship: she was living with her partner of twelve years in an RDP house with their three children. Elaborating on her moral character, Zinzi stated that she would never have a casual partner because such relationships are built only around the exchange of sex and money. Likewise, she had not joined the trial casually. Many women similarly spoke of their trial participation in terms of their strong sense of purpose and intent—one that was voluntary. During a group discussion, a participant noted, "For some of them it is like a job, but we are volunteering." The other women present agreed that they too were volunteers, adding that most participants were interested only in the financial benefits of the trial. Like many others, they stressed that the trial was a way to monitor their health and receive care.

In some instances, women were accosted over their choice to join the trial. A participant recalled, "Some treat me bad—they say I love money and that is why I am participating in the study." Another commented, "My friends are saying that I want to infect them with my gel when I ask them to come and join the study." A third had similar experiences: "People keep on taunting me, saying that I am selling my blood to you [the clinic]. . . . [They ask,] 'Why are you selling your blood?'" In rare cases, accusations led to assault. After leaving the clinic, one participant was confronted by a group of boys yelling at her for selling her blood. They then robbed her of the R150 she had received from the clinic. Consequently, some women chose to hide their participation: "I did not tell anyone about the gel because I thought it is between me and my partner. You know why I don't tell them? It's because they said we are coming here to get AIDS so why must I tell them? Meanwhile, they were saying bad things about the gel and why they take our blood." Community speculation about the trial played a significant role in how women were treated at home and as they went about their daily tasks.

## CRITICAL COMMENTARIES

While not unanticipated, rumors of harm frustrated trial staff, who often dismissed the tales as misinformation or myth. Trialists often assume that any attitudes they consider to be erroneous can be corrected through education. Recognizing that rumors can disrupt medical research, clinical trial programs often include a community participation (or "public engagement") component (Fairhead et al. 2006). To mitigate negative perceptions of the research process for a clinical trial in Tanzania, residents attended practical demonstrations of blood and specimen preparation, which were intended to allay their fears of blood theft (Vallely et al. 2007). Yet, despite repeated attempts by trialists to impart increasingly detailed information, speculation often persists (Pool et al. 2006). Rumors that achieve popular legitimacy can have mixed consequences for clinical trials. In some cases, gossip and complaints may have little impact on participation in clinical trials or adherence to medication (Kaler 2009). In others, they can threaten the success of a trial: a study in Ghana lost a high number of participants because of tales about blood theft (Newton et al. 2009); hostile community protests in Kenya threatened a nutrition study (Geissler 2005a); and allegations prompted by blood taking, body measuring, and even the act of providing study participants with biscuits significantly reduced enrollment in a study in Mozambique (Pool et al. 2006).

Stories of gel dumpers were a particular worry for the MDP301: if enough women were discarding their gels unused, the trial would have a flat result even if PRO 2000/5 was efficacious. Although efforts were made to disseminate "accurate" information and to encourage gel use through community meetings, radio programs, and retention parties, tales of malicious murders and greedy liars persisted. The narratives of harm endured despite these efforts because they reflected the larger concerns of Sowetans and Orange Farmers. Trial rumors were situated within and made sense of broader social and political currents (Campion-Vincent 2002; Kaler 2009). Indeed, truth is not necessarily the most important aspect of rumors for those who spread or hear them (Besnier 1994). In this sense, rumors are critical commentaries on the ways in which these trials impact social relations (Geissler et al. 2008). They are a form of everyday protest, weapons wielded by the powerless against the powerful (Scott 1985). Symptomatic of the problematic relationships between the clinical trial and the trial communities, rumors can be understood as popular resistance to biomedical models of behavior and the hegemony of biomedical constructs (Geissler 2005b; Newton et al. 2009; White 2000).

Given that many international trials are now conducted in postcolonial states, the "long conversation" between colonizers and colonized has been continued through medical testing (Comaroff and Comaroff 1991). Thaba noted that he was initially suspicious of "white people's stuff," particularly medical interventions, because of the conspicuous injustices black people had suffered in South Africa. When those spearheading education campaigns and interventions appear to be wealthy, white, and foreign, narratives of white malice, contaminated pharmaceuticals, and blood selling are made much more meaningful and credible (Geissler 2005a; Kaler 2009; Niehaus and Jonsson 2005). Tales of Basson or the CIA creating HIV as a biological weapon reflect a suspicion resulting from a long history of white oppression in South Africa. Similarly, stories of coffin money and blood selling couple historical relationships with everyday observations, associating cash with injurious and exploitative procedures. Emphasizing the stark difference between the people employed by the trial and the ordinary participants, these narratives reconfigure the relationship between researchers and researched by constructing a counter-epistemic commentary through which historical and contemporary relationships between "poor Africans" and "wealthy whites" can be expressed and critiqued. Examining rumors of organ stealing, Nancy Scheper-Hughes (1996:9) wrote, "The stories are told, remembered, and circulated because they are fundamentally, *existentially* true." Bracketed by a continuing history of inequality, economic domination, and repressive public health, Soweto and Orange Farm residents expressed a genuine reality—black people were disproportionately suffering the effects of AIDS, clinical trials had been proven hazardous, and trial doctors did drive expensive vehicles.

Responses to the MDP301 and other clinical trials embody the deep personal, economic, and social anxieties that pervade the postcolonial world. Soweto and Orange Farm have experienced histories of segregation, disenfranchisement, and continued poverty. Despite the end of apartheid and the promises of many black politicians, the fortunes of most Sowetans and Orange Farmers such as Thaba have not improved. In seeking explanations, South Africans have increasingly focused on the prevalence of witchcraft. Since the apartheid era, anthropologists have documented a rise in "spiritual insecurities" (Ashforth 2005) and "occult economies" (Comaroff and Comaroff 2000; Comaroff and Comaroff 1999), in which harmful magic is employed to achieve monetary benefit. Exemplifying this trend, witchcraft is an acute source of concern throughout the nation. Functioning as much more than a system of explanation, witchcraft represents a fundamental threat to the social and moral structure of society (White 2000).

In South Africa, the idiom of witchcraft has undergone significant transformations, reflecting changes in the political economy. Historical narratives stress the inherited ability to perform witchcraft, which flows through breast milk from mother to child, and an accumulation of secret knowledge. Dangerous to all, witches also use their magical powers to punish criminals and avenge victims of wrongdoing. They harness their skills from the natural world—the lightning bird can manipulate electrical storms, and magical medicine (isiZulu: *muthi*) is dug up and plucked from the forests. In the postcolonial and apartheid eras, witchcraft became commoditized: magical substances are easily procured through newspaper ads promising boundless wealth and beautiful women, while witch familiars include the *mamlambo* (isiZulu), a snakelike creature that transforms into a white woman who requires the sacrifice of kinsmen's blood in exchange for cash. Users of witchcraft are thought to be motivated by greed and envy, while victims of witchcraft, the undead, are exploited by witches to labor on their farms and factories. These transformations reveal a sharp critique of the contemporary political economy, in which commodities and cash have eroded ties of kinship and sociability (Niehaus 2001). Sharing many of the motifs found in witchcraft accounts, tales of clinical trials and other medical interactions likewise provide a series of narratives through which spiritual insecurities are similarly negotiated.

Analogous to rumors about the MDP301, the immoral exchange of blood for wealth and the misfortune that results from it are recurring themes in witchcraft narratives. Witches are accused of deviously taking innocent people's blood, giving it to familiars, and receiving cash in exchange (Bähre 2002). Although money is gained through these transactions, it is portrayed as "unproductive and sterile," failing to benefit the wider society (Niehaus 2000:50). These illicit exchanges threaten the very fabric of family and sociality. While blood is considered a vital bodily fluid, it also embodies notions of personhood. Conceptualized as the comingling of a man's white blood and a woman's red blood, the transfer of fluids during sexual intercourse is essential to the constitution of individuals and their relationships to one another (Thornton 2008). These exchanges acquire social legitimacy through the payment of *lobola*, which is given for a woman's "blood" or reproductive potential. In this way, blood and cash are necessary components of ensuring social continuity. If these transactions are perverted or hijacked—for instance, when blood is stolen for profit—the foundation of society is put at risk.

Incorporating the MDP301, its staff, and medical procedures into these long-standing narratives, spiritual anxieties formed the bedrock of accounts regarding coffin money, blood selling, and contaminated gels. Thaba reported that a close friend, whom he had grown up with in a rural homeland, had linked the trial to witchcraft:

*Thaba*: When [my friend] discovered that his partner was participating in this clinic he thought it was witchcraft. He scolded the woman, saying she is bringing white people's witchcraft in his house.

*Interviewer*: Why did he think it was witchcraft?

*Thaba*: He said white people are bewitching them; they have put other people's sperms in the applicator and the woman inserts them inside her vagina so when a man has sex with the woman they do so on top of the other person's sperms.

*Interviewer*: What did his partner say when she was scolded?

*Thaba*: They discussed together and then my friend came over to me and said, "You know what, my friend, my partner is attending that clinic and they give them sperms to insert in their vaginas before we could have sex and she has been using their things for a while now and she has never told me."

In these statements, the alleged presence of foreign sperm in the gel endangers a legitimate exchange between Africans, thereby undermining their heritage. Other community members noted the similarity between narratives of witches stealing blood and trial administrators selling blood.[12] We were told that trial staff resembled witches "thirsty for their own child's blood" and that blood draws proved that the trial staff was engaging in witchcraft.[13] Not only do these statements stress the oppression of Africans by foreign powers, they do so by invoking representations of an irreplaceable and priceless resource—lifeblood—without which health, self, and procreation would collapse (Saethre and Stadler 2013). Because wealth obtained at the expense of social reproduction can lead only to death, trial participants were said to buy their coffins.

Trial narratives not only reflected notions about relationships between white researchers and black subjects, but also formed part of a larger conversation about gender in Orange Farm and Soweto. Since the 1970s, sub-Saharan Africans have expressed concern over both the growing independence of urban women and the link between sexual relationships and monetary ones (Cornwall 2002; Kaler 2006; Wojcicki 2002a; Wojcicki 2002b). As the men of Soweto and Orange Farm attempt to save *lobola* to start a family, women increasingly access cash through state welfare payments and transactional sex. Stories of greedy women and gel dumpers mirrored widespread assumptions—affirmed by both men and women—that cast young women as using either the state or men as an "easy" means of accessing cash. Discussing the high prevalence of women engaging in transactional sex, one participant noted, "Other women do tell us that they are not in love with their partners; they just want money." This perspective was elaborated on by another woman:

> When they see money they pretend as if they love. Meanwhile, there is no love. . . . Yes, there is someone who has a boyfriend that has money and she loves him because he has money. There are people who are close to that person and they tell you that he has money and he can give you money. You find that she does not love the guy but she wants his money. She even says he is ugly but he has money.

The desire for cash was thought to motivate women to engage in premarital sex with a variety of partners instead of remaining virgins until their wedding nights. One individual told us, "I think for men to give women money makes them sleep around because they have this thing that the more partners they have the more they will make money." Once married, wives could be prompted either to deceive or divorce their husbands in the hope of gaining greater resources from another man. A male resident commented, "You find women, when a man does not give them more money they break up with that man and then find someone who is going to give them more money."

During a focus group discussion with four women from Orange Farm, they all condemned "selling your body" as immoral and stressed that it resulted in promiscuity and infidelity. The women contrasted this with *lobola*, which was "good" because it demonstrated that "your parents looked after you." Whereas *lobola* cemented procreative relationships, money gained from feigning love was thought to profit the individual rather than the collective. Women were said to purchase commodities such as fashionable clothes or perfumes for their sole use. Associated exclusively with the female gender, these items did not, and could not, benefit the entire family. Money acquired via sex was often depicted as a threat to 'traditional" gender and family relations. Consequently, statements condemning women for using sex to access cash were not confined to males. Acting as a force that is "expressive and transformative" (Cornwall 2002:971), commoditized relationships rearticulate and reshape gender and family interactions.

Given the convergence of female participants, sexual activity, and cash reimbursements, the MDP301 became incorporated into existing gender dialogues. Not only could gel use be concealed from men, so could the money resulting from trial participation: "The study gives me money. He doesn't have to know anything about that money. It is my money." Another participant agreed: "The money—no, I didn't think it was important to tell him about the money." Framed by a wider unease regarding women's access to undisclosed money via premarital sexual relationships, participation in the trial became a focus around which these notions were expressed. In many instances, the MDP301 seemed to assume the characteristics of an illicit male lover—one who provided women with clandestine income but who could also be deceived. Interestingly, women were said to dump the gel in the long grass, where affairs are thought to be conducted. Greedy participants were accused of "playing with" RHRU, much as they did with their boyfriends. Instead of feigning love or hiding infidelity, trial participants cheated by dumping the gel and lying to clinic staff, and then boasted to friends about the deception. A participant described a waiting-room conversation in which another woman had bragged about discarding the contents of five applicators and about how the trial staff would never know. This conversation resembled others between women about their clueless ATM boyfriends. Furthermore, discarding the gel, like engaging in transactional sex, was portrayed as benefiting the individual: dumpers were accused of purchasing "fashionable clothes" with the money they obtained from the trial. In addition, these participants were charged with placing the success of the trial at risk and threatening the development of a pharmaceutical that could conceivably benefit millions of African women. Through these accounts, the MDP301 was transformed into a vehicle for conveying local gender concerns regarding who should be having sex and for what reasons.

In some ways, microbicide technology itself encouraged community members to create signification. In a setting where HIV risk is often equated with multipartner sex, microbicides can appear to be a technology for promiscuous women. Not only do microbicides seem to transgress sexual norms, their ability to be hidden also overtly restructures gender relations. Introduced to support female autonomy in HIV prevention, microbicides were designed as a tool that could be used without the tacit knowledge of a sexual partner. Assuming that some women would choose to conceal their utilization of a microbicide gel, the MDP301 did not require participants to inform their partners of their enrollment or the money they received. Cash reimbursements gave women an independent source of income that could be hidden from their partners. Consequently, it is hardly surprising that the trial became a locus around which narratives of women's agency were debated.

While the MDP301 was successful in providing women with pharmaceuticals and reimbursements that could be concealed from men, in so doing, it ignited fears that gender relations and social reproduction would be fundamentally challenged. As a result, young women on the trial were not only the subject of rumors, but occasionally verbally confronted by friends, family, and even strangers if they were seen going to the clinic.

Considering that microbicide technology was developed to aid young unmarried women, it is ironic that the residents of Orange Farm and Soweto often equated sincere trial participation with stable sexual relationships and disclosure to partners. The women whom microbicides were supposed to empower the most were those accused of dumping their gels and lying to the trial. Despite the messages of the trial, participants and community members made their own interpretation of what was occurring. Through rumors of malicious trialists selling blood and greedy women dumping their gels, the MDP301 was situated within local frameworks of meaning. As narratives about the MDP301 circulated through Soweto and Orange Farm, the trial ceased to be a strictly foreign enterprise. Instead of standing apart from community narratives, the MDP301 was incorporated into them by raising deep-seated questions about the morality of young women's conduct and in particular their use of their bodies for self-enrichment. Through the process of witnessing, discussing, and participating in the trial, Sowetans and Orange Farmers fashioned the MDP301 into a tool through which ongoing social processes and insecurities were affirmed, debated, and contested.

# Libidinous
# Sociality

Echoing colonial narratives that dwelled on the aberrance and exoticness of African sexual behaviors, public health research contends that many sub-Saharan Africans prefer to engage in what is popularly known as dry sex (Beksinska et al. 1999; Civic and Wilson 1996; Hull et al. 2011). Those participating in dry sex purportedly eschew any form of vaginal lubrication or moisture, believing that the practice grants men greater pleasure while confirming the virtuousness of women. Given the assumed ubiquity and intractability of the dry sex ideal, a number of researchers have questioned if a microbicide suspended in a lubricating medium will be accepted by African women (Bagnol and Mariano 2008; Beksinska et al. 1999; Kun 1998; Scorgie et al. 2009). Attempting to gauge if PRO 2000/5 would be embraced or rejected by those using it, MDP301 coordinators sought to understand couples' sexual experiences with the gel. In an effort to easily characterize participant's reactions, trial coordinators constructed rubrics of statistically analyzable dichotomies such as wet/dry and acceptable/unacceptable. However, these clinical categories failed to convey the complexity of women's sexual lives and struggles.

Anxiety about STIs, infidelity, or violence could quickly transform sex into a stressful or even painful act. Kagiso, for instance, lived in fear that one day she would contract AIDS. As a 45-year-old woman, she had seen many people die of what she assumed was AIDS and was desperate to avoid that fate. Although she had been faithful to her second husband of five years, she was unsure about his fidelity. He worked as a minibus taxi driver and spent every Friday night drinking at informal bars in Orange Farm, not returning home until Saturday morning. Although he claimed to be staying with his parents, Kagiso suspected that he was engaging in transactional sex with young women wishing to "fundraise." She tried to insist on condom usage but her husband refused, saying they caused him pain and bloating. Kagiso was particularly frustrated because he was a "Zulu man" and spoke about something only when he disliked it. They argued about his absences and excuses but nothing changed. When Kagiso could not stop feeling cold one summer, she convinced herself that she had become HIV positive. Relieved that her HIV test was negative, Kagiso joined the MDP301, only to discover that she had contracted genital herpes from her husband.

Like Kagiso, Zanele also viewed sex with trepidation. Zanele was unemployed and considered herself a housewife. She had been with her partner for 16 years and they had one child together. Although wedding rings had not been exchanged, he had paid *lobola*. Zanele said that like many couples, they fought about small things, like smoking in the house. Even though they had disagreements and she occasionally threatened to leave him, Zanele believed that their relationship was stable and "all right": he was understanding, didn't force her to have sex, and used a condom if she asked him to. After Zanele's second pregnancy ended in the premature birth and death of that child, she had tried to get pregnant once again. But despite their long time together and desire to have more children, Zanele was always nervous about having sex with her partner, particularly if the lights were turned on. As a result, she was seldom able to get aroused and the lack of lubrication made sex painful. Zanele confessed that her anxiety had begun at the age of 17, when her stepfather had almost raped her. Although her sister had interrupted them before he could penetrate her, Zanele was extremely traumatized. Every time she began to have sex, the episode came into her mind.

Women like Kagiso and Zanele are not alone. Across South Africa and around the world, women are victims of rape and sexual intimidation. Even in so-called good relationships, women often have little say over sexual matters. Consequently, feminist scholars—noting that social norms surrounding sex prioritize male pleasure while penalizing women more than men for transgressions—tend to view sex as a primary method through which men are able to control and ultimately exploit women (LeMoncheck 1997). Assumptions regarding women's powerlessness, coupled with data demonstrating women's inability to insist on condom use in sub-Saharan Africa, have spurred the development of microbicides. Beyond the creation of medical technology, these perspectives also constrain notions of Africanness. Ifi Amadiume (2006:27) notes that casting men as the sole sexual agent "simply restates and reinforces the perspective and practice of male power over female sexuality and this is not the whole story of sexuality in Africa."

While sub-Saharan African women's sexual behaviors, particularly in the context of HIV/AIDS, have received a great deal of attention, their sexual agency and pleasure have been largely ignored (Spronk 2005; Skafte and Silberschmidt 2014; Tamale 2011). Although sex can serve as a tool of female oppression, it can also precipitate female liberation. Through sexual gratification, women are able to transform themselves from sexual objects to sexual subjects and contest the power of men.

While Kagiso and Zanele had enrolled in the trial to monitor their health, they quickly discovered that the gel had a profound effect on their sex lives. Both women began enjoying sex much more and engaging in it more frequently. They, along with many other women, believed that the gel acted as an aphrodisiac. Almost half (47 percent) of the participants who rated the gel as highly "acceptable" in in-depth interviews also said that it increased sexual enjoyment. Instead of inserting drying agents into their vaginas to improve their sex lives, participants began using the gel. Despite trialists' fears that the gel would be universally condemned for its wetness, it was instead praised for its ability to magnify pleasure during sex. Shaped by social expectations as well as everyday experiences, the women's perception of the gel evolved, transforming it from a potential HIV prevention tool into a sexual aid that fundamentally altered relationships. Satisfied with the sex he was having with his wife, Kagiso's husband no longer spent nights away from home. Able to achieve orgasms easily for the first time, Zanele had the confidence to be honest with her partner about her sexual feelings. Earlier, she had "felt ashamed," but after joining the MDP301, she had become "able to ask him questions like how he felt during sex and he answers me; we are able to communicate about sex." As participants and their partners noted that improved sex resulted in improved relationships, women like Zanele invoked their own gendered agency more often. Through sexual pleasure, the gel and the trial reshaped female sociality.

## WET AND DRY

Around the globe, a variety of vaginal insertion practices have been observed (Hull et al. 2011). These habits, as well as the normative ideals that underpin them, were researched sporadically throughout the mid-twentieth century. With the advent of HIV/AIDS, what had previously been regarded as a scholarly curiosity became a topic of international interest. Seeking to explain the disproportionate rates of HIV infection in sub-Saharan Africa, researchers seized on the notion of culture. By the mid-1980s, a number of scholars were cataloging a range of so-called African practices that were dubbed high-risk behaviors. In 1988, it was suggested that the intravaginal insertion of drying substances by female sex workers in Zaire (present-day Democratic Republic of the Congo) placed them in considerably greater jeopardy of contracting HIV (Mann et al. 1988). There was a concern that moisture-reducing agents could disrupt the integrity of the vaginal epithelium, making it more prone to abrasion and tearing during sexual intercourse. Researchers hypothesized that if the vaginal lining was compromised, this would eliminate an important barrier to the virus entering the bloodstream. As articles focusing on the link between vaginal practices and African culture were published throughout the 1990s, dry sex was almost universally portrayed as dangerous (Brown et al. 1993; Runganga and Kasule 1995; van de Wijgert et al. 1999).[1] As further investigations were conducted over the years, the link between dry sex and AIDS was challenged. Although some researchers continue to assert that the use of vaginal drying agents is a risk factor for contracting HIV, to date there is no conclusive evidence to support this assumption (Levin 2005; Morar et al. 2003; Myer et al. 2005; Reddy et al. 2009).

Research has confirmed that across much of continent, Africans state that the vagina should be dry, tight, and warm prior to intercourse (Bagnol and Mariano 2008; Beksinska et al. 1999; Civic and Wilson 1996; Gafos et al. 2010; Scorgie et al. 2009).[2] While the early literature assumed women's notions of dryness meant a complete lack of vaginal moisture, recent studies indicate that a more realistic interpretation is an absence of excessive wetness (Scorgie et al. 2009). If vaginal fluids cause noise to be produced during intercourse, for example, women often feel embarrassed for being too wet. In addition to dryness, tightness and warmth appear to be equally important vaginal characteristics. To create these qualities, women inserted a variety of substances, including household detergents, patent medicines, antiseptics, and locally produced herbal remedies. These products are said to be employed by women for two primary purposes: as a means of concealing sexual transgressions, and to ensure that a man remains sexually interested in his partner (Gafos et al. 2010; Scorgie et al. 2009). MDP301 doctors hypothesized that the presence of these materials could potentially alter the chemical effectiveness of PRO 2000/5. Consequently, the trial attempted to catalogue the beliefs and practices surrounding dry sex and intravaginal insertion comprehensively (Allen et al. 2010).[3]

Women in Johannesburg reported that dry and tight vaginas were often praised and described as "like a child's." One participant confided that a close friend had told her, "When you want to be like this [shows a closed fist], you must use snuff. Snuff takes your vagina back to the way it was initially."[4] Many women, including Tshepiso, Nomsa, Andiswa, Zanele, and Boikanyo, confirmed that snuff was used intravaginally. Zinzi recalled seeing a neighbor buy the product but never chew it: "One of my friends told me that this lady doesn't inhale it, but she inserts it in the vagina. We asked her why she was doing that. She said that she doesn't want her partner to run away from her." Another woman remarked, "Snuff is hot so when it gets to the vagina it makes it dry." While snuff was the most popular product mentioned, other materials were also used. Drying and tightening agents included baby oil, Vicks VapoRub, Zam-Buk (an ointment used to soothe cuts, sores, and insect bites), Disperin (soluble aspirin), vinegar, Dettol (liquid antiseptic), lemon juice, brown paper, and ice. Other women sought to avoid products purported to make their vaginas wet, such as coffee and caffeine. In one instance, sliced cucumbers were said to be inserted vaginally to achieve the same toning effect that occurred when they were placed on the eyes. Not only were youthful faces deemed attractive, so too were youthful vaginas.

Because arousal and intercourse were believed to alter a woman's body, vaginal state was seen as an important indicator of female sexual activity. A survey conducted in Orange Farm reported that the main reason dryness was preferred was that it demonstrated a lack of promiscuity (Beksinska et al. 1999). Women who engaged in sex frequently and with a number of men were thought to have noticeably wet and loose vaginas. Boikanyo noted, "When you don't use condoms all the time, the vagina becomes too wet. It is worse when you have multiple partners. . . . When you are sleeping with too many men, the vagina develops a smell as well. But when you are committed to one partner, there will be no need for you to use [drying agents] and all those things because your vagina will not have any of those problems." Men often reported monitoring the vaginal state of their partners as a way of determining fidelity. Tebogo stated, "You see, most of us men, we have a belief that when you have sex with your partner we expect her to be tight. She cannot be loose. She has to grip you or else you start to suspect that she is cheating." Acutely aware that men equated the state of their vagina with the state of their faithfulness, women were particularly concerned about how partners perceived their bodies. Both men and women reported that one of the primary reasons women used substances vaginally was to hide sexual indiscretions. Inserting a drying and tightening agent after having intercourse with one partner, a woman could immediately visit another who would have no way of physically determining that she was unfaithful. Boikanyo, who stressed that she had never used products such as snuff, concluded, "I think inserting things in the vagina is common among promiscuous women who have sex with multiple partners, because they don't want the other partner to realize that they are having sex with another man." Women accused of using drying agents in this manner were often cast as immoral, manipulating their partners for financial gain.

Whereas drying agents could be used to conceal indiscretions, they were also a tool to ensure male fidelity through sexual pleasure. A dry, tight, and warm vagina was thought to increase friction and consequently male arousal. Women who used intravaginal products were said to stimulate men in a way that others could not. Zanele said, "They want to increase the taste, like being enjoyable or increasing the passion they feel during sex." It was assumed that once a man was sexually satisfied, he would not engage in affairs outside the relationship. One woman noted that if a woman inserted snuff prior to intercourse "when her partner has sex with another woman he does not feel the same as when he has sex with her." Unable to experience an equivalent level of enjoyment, he would abandon any thought of having a mistress. Many other women echoed these views. One summed them up: "These things that they insert, some women do it so that they can possess a man. They . . . get something that can make a man to feel all the heat and pleasure of sex so that he does not leave her." She added that this way the man would "love only her."[5]

The main motivations for women practicing intravaginal insertion include the perceptions and desires of men. Sowetans and Orange Farmers often stressed that male enjoyment was possible only if there was friction between the penis and vagina. Reproductive health research has also found that women report participating in dry sex mainly to satisfy their partners and increase male pleasure (Beksinska et al. 1999; Brown and Brown 2000; Morar et al. 2003; Myer et al. 2005; Reddy et al. 2009). While these responses have been viewed as a consequence of male dominance in sexual realms (Levin 2005; Scorgie et al. 2009), this is only one factor in women's decisions. Noting that their survey revealed sexually inactive women were also using drying agents, Mbololwa Mbikusita-Lewanika et al. (2009:237) conclude that vaginal state was intimately "related to the whole concept of womanhood, societal expectations, and self-image." Despite the importance of male preferences, vaginal insertion practices are also grounded in female notions of femininity.

Equated with achieving the virginal ideal, tightness is associated with purity (Hilber et al. 2012:1319; Scorgie et al. 2009:281) and a woman's moral constitution (Leclerc-Madlala 2001b). Practices such as the use of drying agents and the elongation of the labia minora actively mold a woman's body, creating a successful space for procreation and social reproduction. Women demonstrate that they are ready for womanhood, sex, and a stable family by working to attain their social position (Hilber et al. 2012:1319). Furthermore, fashioning a dry, tight, and warm vagina expresses a desire to have a long-term love relationship and "hold onto a man" (Bagnol and Mariano 2008:577; Scorgie et al. 2009:278). Capturing a man's sexual devotion ensures a stable relationship, rather than one in which a man spends money on other women (threatening financial well-being) or contracts sexually transmitted infections (threatening physical well-being). As a locus for drying agents and love medicines, the vagina becomes a tool to express not only female aspirations but also power. While men often dominate sexual encounters—for instance, by determining the frequency of sex and condom use—narratives of dry sex articulate female agency over men by stressing women's ability to control male desire and capture their devotion (Scorgie et al. 2009:280).

To understand the significance behind narratives of dry and tight sex, we must not only situate vaginal insertion practices within a larger sociocultural framework of meaning but also supplement these meanings with the experiences of women and the way in which these practices are lived on a daily basis. Studies conducted in Zambia (Mbikusita-Lewanika et al. 2009) and South Africa (Gafos et al. 2010; Morar et al. 2003; Reddy et al. 2009) have shown that while almost all the women interviewed were aware of vaginal insertion practices, rates of use varied considerably. While 141 of 150 (94 percent) sex workers in KwaZulu-Natal inserted substances to achieve dry sex (Morar et al. 2003:371), only 159 of 446 (36.72 percent) women surveyed in the Western Cape stated that they preferred dry sex (Reddy et al. 2009:79). Furthermore, research has shown that women can find dry sex extremely uncomfortable (Morar et al. 2003). Brigitte Bagnol and Esmeralda

Mariano (2008) assert that while the actual experience of dry sex is often painful, it is nevertheless the ideal. They write, "Lacerations on the penis and in the vagina are reported as a consequence of the effort needed to penetrate and the friction. For these men and women, it is often not possible to separate perceived pleasure and pain in the context of sexual intercourse. The difficulty of penetration, the tightness and the dryness of the vagina are considered to be the most valuable forms of sexual enjoyment" (581).

There has been a tendency to view Africans as simply putting up with the discomfort of dry sex, despite abrasions and other difficulties, either to please men or enact social meaning. But, contrary to the findings of some researchers, women in Johannesburg were extremely hesitant to insert drying and tightening substances vaginally, despite the social and cultural meanings attached to the act. Although we collected many secondhand tales of vaginal insertion practices, few women described personally engaging in them. Of the 150 women interviewed, only 4 stated that they had inserted a vaginal drying substance (in their cases, either Dettol or snuff).[6] While most women said that they did not use drying substances, they simultaneously added that many of their friends, neighbors, acquaintances, and friends of friends did. We suspect that if women were indeed inserting vaginal substances at the rate rumored, we would have received more firsthand reports from the MDP301 participants. Although this discrepancy could be explained in terms of women choosing to conceal their vaginal practices for fear of being labeled promiscuous, our interview data suggests that this was not the case.

In conversations with trial participants and community members, we were repeatedly told that apprehension over discomfort, illness, and toxicity discouraged individuals from inserting substances vaginally. Neither Zinzi, Mothudi, Nomsa, Andiswa, Zanele, nor Boikanyo had ever used drying substances. Women worried that materials such as snuff or Dispirin would cause vaginal pain or burning sensations. Referring to her choice to abstain from using drying agents, Zanele commented, "I don't think it's necessary because God made us the way we are. These things are dangerous. For example, snuff causes cancer and putting it inside the vagina is risky and the vagina is sensitive." Women asked why they should take these risks when dry sex was not a practice they believed they would enjoy. Several participants commented that a small and dry vagina would actually make sex difficult and painful, if not impossible. One asked, "How can you have sex when you are completely dry?" Reflecting on her own experiences, Zanele said, "Dry sex is painful and I don't know why people would want to have that." Other women asserted that they had no need to have dry sex because their partners were already satisfied with their sexual performance. Boikanyo commented, "I have not heard any of my partners tell me that I am not hot in bed, so I don't see the point of inserting things in my vagina." These statements highlight a pervasive slippage between the social meanings attached to a dry and tight vagina and the everyday realities of sexual relations. On one hand, dry sex narratives remain popular because they portray an idealized version of femininity, in which women are able to assert their virtue and agency through their vaginas. On the other hand, anxiety about pain and illness discouraged women from actually engaging in dry sex practices.

## FROM EXPERIMENTAL PHARMACEUTICAL TO APHRODISIAC

Concerns regarding the comfort and safety of drying and tightening products were mirrored in women's initial reactions to the trial gel. Worries about discomfort and health consequences were frequently mentioned in discussions with potential participants. However, several women altered their views and enrolled, in part because the trial was demonstrably controlled and sanctioned by doctors. Interestingly, increased wetness was not one of the fears expressed by participants prior to gel use. Given that the gel ostensibly functioned as a lubricant, trial coordinators wondered if participants would find it too wet and intolerable. Indeed, this was the case for some women. Thandiwe noted, "Since I started using the gel, I started realizing changes in my body because the gel made me to be wet." For Thandiwe and others like her, this experience was unacceptable. But as the trial progressed, women's perceptions of the gel shifted. Thandiwe was so worried about the wetness she was experiencing that she consulted a friend who was also participating in the trial: "She told me to continue using it: once it gets used to you, you will no longer notice the wetness. I followed her advice and felt that I am right. I'm no longer wet; I'm the way I used to be." Examining responses such as this, it is clear that the distinction between wet and dry was more complex than researchers had anticipated. Rather than branding the gel as fundamentally wet, women's opinions differed dramatically. While some asserted that the gel made their vaginas wet, others claimed that it had a drying effect. In focus groups, it was not uncommon to have one participant vociferously proclaim that the gel caused wetness while another declared that it dried her vagina. In some cases, the gel could be viewed as having both properties concurrently. Reflecting on the changes in his partner's body, Hendrick remarked, "The gel makes her vagina moist enough that she does not feel any pain but also a bit dry so that sex is still enjoyable." These differences of opinion led to debates in which neither side altered their views. Instead, it was acknowledged that the gel's properties were different for each woman.

Diverging from the trial's expectations, several women, including Zinzi, commented that the gel dried their vaginas. Many of these individuals noted that prior to joining the trial, wetness had been a significant problem. One woman commented, "I see a lot of changes [from using the gel]. Before, I used to be very wet when I was about to have sex with my partner, but now that I am using the gel I feel very dry inside." A married participant had a similar experience: "A woman can be a little wet down there, so he [her husband] said that since I have used the gel I am dry and I feel so nice." She described this feeling as "just dry, but not too dry." Participants stressed not only the drying properties of the gel but also its ability to reduce vaginal size and increase heat. Just as snuff was credited with making the vagina tight and youthful, so too was the gel. Kagiso reported, "The gel makes the vagina tight and it becomes like that of a child." Echoing this perspective, one participant said simply, "[The gel] makes me feel like I am a virgin again."

Several women noted that the gel also increased vaginal warmth, referring to it as "a fire." Busi commented, "I feel very good when I have used the gel because it makes me hot and it has brought back my sex life and I just feel like a young girl. I am very grateful for the gel because I really enjoy using it." For these women, the gel acted similarly to drying and tightening substances. In some cases, male partners mistook the effects of the gel for those of other products. Busi recounted how the experience of having sex after she had inserted the gel had led her partner to believe that she was using a substance such as snuff:

> He is feeling good about the gel because he asked what happened because he felt that I was different and I told him that I had used the gel. He even commented that he feels that I am so hot now and he wondered if I had inserted something [a drying and tightening product]. And I told him that I had inserted the gel only. He thought I was inserting other things that people use but I told him I had inserted the gel and that is all I am using.

These women and their partners praised the gel for its drying, tightening, and warming properties while remarking that their experiences of sexual intercourse were greatly improved.

Another group of participants claimed that the gel produced wetness and described it as making vaginas smooth, moist, and lubricated. Several women reported that, prior to joining the trial, they had felt too dry during sex, describing their vaginal skin as cracked or desiccated. As a result, vaginal penetration had been uncomfortable or painful. Lubricants had not been used and concerns over infected condoms had led some men to wipe off any emollient prior to intercourse. As a result, sex had been painful. Boikanyo noted, "I had a problem that I struggled with for a very long time. I used to get cuts on my vagina when I had sex and this made sex in general very unpleasant for me. But with the gel, it is easier for my partner to penetrate me and I don't get cuts anymore." For other women, dryness had been the result of a lack of foreplay. Goitsemedime said that because her partner is often away working, "when he returns home you find that he has the strong desire to have sex, such that he cannot wait for foreplay. Sometimes we try to have foreplay but he will be in a hurry and the foreplay becomes short because he is in a hurry to have sex. And when we have sex, I am not yet ready." During past reunions, "he had to force his penis into my vagina and it was painful." As a result, "sometimes he would just stop and could not have sex because it was painful for me." But after using the gel for the first time, Goitsemedime discovered that "penetration was easy and I did not feel pain anymore. I enjoyed sex more than before and my partner liked it because I was no longer feeling pain during sex. I was not screaming anymore." In instances such as these, lubrication was not viewed as an indication of promiscuity or thought to precipitate male sexual dissatisfaction. Rather, it was viewed as a welcome alternative to uncomfortable sex.

Whether they perceived the gel as a cause of wetness or dryness, most women asserted that it improved their sexual encounters and radically increased enjoyment.[7] Women described experiencing greater vaginal and sexual sensitivity, noting that they had "more feelings" while using the gel. Nomsa observed, "It is different from before because when we have sex I get more excited." These new sensations produced effortless and frequent arousal. Zanele said, "I had the problem of taking time to be aroused, but when I started using the gel all that changed." Like Zanele, Pretty noted, "Before [using the gel] he used to finish before me. When I use the gel and then we start to have sex, I orgasm quickly, but before I used to take a long time to orgasm." Other women described routinely experiencing multiple orgasms for the first time. In all these cases, the gel was credited. Thandi described the changes in sexual arousal as follows: "The difference was, you know, before I did not feel my man in that way or enjoy what we were doing. But since I started using the gel, you know, I feel that I am having sex with . . . my boyfriend and I am enjoying everything, you know. Yes, I think that is the difference. The gel brought me . . . the pleasure of having sex." Citing intense feelings of arousal, another participant remarked that the gel made her high during sex. Comments such as these were echoed by a significant number of participants. Women were amazed to discover that they were relishing sex appreciably more than they had previously.

This newfound enjoyment altered the attitudes and practices of women toward sex. Many participants said that prior to joining the trial the discomfort associated with sex made them and their partners tired, weary, and disinterested. As a result, women routinely attempted to minimize sexual activities or avoid them altogether. Another participant commented, "Before I started using the gel I was pretending and it was difficult to say to my partner that I don't want to have sex because he is not always at home. Have you ever noticed how painful it is, pretending to enjoy sex when you are not enjoying it at all?" However, after joining the trial, she noticed dramatic changes in her sexual responses: "Since I started the gel things are totally different. I'm now active and eager to have sex." Lerato had a similar experience. She remarked, "When you have sex with your partner it is like you do not become tired. It [the gel] makes me want to have sex all the time." Many other women in the trial also noted that their earlier experiences of fatigue during sex had disappeared. Thandiwe reported, "This gel made other changes in me. I was too lazy to have sex, but nowadays I am the one who initiates sex. The minute he arrives I'm all over him. It's like this gel has opened something that has been closed in me. I like the gel so much." Rather than draining their energy, sex now invigorated women.

As a result, women reported desiring and engaging in sex much more frequently and energetically. One participant told us that she and other women in the trial "never used to enjoy sex," but, with the gel, they wanted to have sex with their partners "all the time." Andiswa noted that previously she had been content to abstain from sex for four or more days at a time, but since she began using the gel, this was no longer possible. For many couples, having sex more often also entailed having several sequential episodes or rounds. Boikanyo observed that, before the trial, she "wouldn't want to go on to the second round because already my vagina would be feeling hot and painful," but now she looked forward to having several rounds. Noting that her enjoyment of sex and her sex drive had both increased dramatically, Kagiso added, "In the past we used to have one sex act and then sleep but now we have at least two or even three rounds and I think it is because of the gel." The freedom to have and enjoy multiple sexual acts was described as liberating. A participant asserted that "I don't have to worry if my partner wants to have a second round. I don't have to worry about the pain during penetration. I used to feel sex was a burden because I was uncomfortable to have a second round. Now it is more fun because I know that I will insert the gel and have the second and the third round. Who knows? Maybe I will get introduced to the fourth round!" No longer fearful of discomfort or pain, participants relished their sexual encounters. This motivated some couples to attempt new sexual techniques. Discussing the new positions she achieved with her partner while on the gel, Nqobile said, "It is just that it made me to be flexible when it came to sex. We would do it all the time and I was always right. I didn't feel any pain when I used it. I was so flexible, really." Women were not only enjoying sex but also actively prolonging sexual encounters, increasing their frequency, and performing sex in novel ways.

Discerning a conspicuous shift in participants' behavior during sex, men commented that their partners were now more active and energetic. For women who failed to disclose their trial participation, these changes were sometimes difficult to explain. Thaba's partner, Precious, did not initially inform him of her gel use. However, after she began enjoying having as many as six rounds, Thaba asked her if she was taking a "booster" or aphrodisiac. While Precious disclosed her participation when confronted by Thaba, not all women did. Another participant recounted, "I'm using it secretly and he has not noticed that I'm using it. He only notices that now I'm active sexually and enjoying sex and he asks me what makes me like that." While a minority of women did not disclose their participation at any point during their enrollment, many others informed their partners prior to joining the trial, or within a few months after they enrolled. In these cases, men tended to echo the views of their partners, crediting the gel with facilitating female sexual enjoyment, arousal, and orgasm. Thaba commented, "Before using the gel she was holding back but now there is a lot of difference; she is more willing and giving her all to our lovemaking. I love making love to my woman." He added, "It is so cool."

Like Thaba, other men found that female enjoyment increased their own pleasure during sex. For some men, this was a result of being able to please their partner sexually. For others, the gel was said to enhance male physical responses. Male partners described having heightened sensations in their penises as well as feeling more stimulated and aroused. A few men stated that the gel eliminated previous sexual dysfunction, allowing them to engage in sex for longer periods. Hendrick said, "I don't ejaculate prematurely anymore and that gives her enough time to enjoy herself as well. When I used to ejaculate too quickly, she would also get bored. But now I can ensure that she is satisfied." Hendrick's partner of four years, Andiswa, noted that while he didn't always verbalize his newfound enjoyment, "his actions say it all." Other women echoed this statement. Boikanyo commented, "I think his actions say it all because now he spends more time on top of me than he did before and when he reaches a climax, you can tell that he is really enjoying what he is doing." Zinzi was also acutely aware of the changes in her partner's sexual behavior: "I can see how happy my partner is and I feel he is more satisfied as a result of the gel. Sex is not the same way it was before even for him."

Men and women noted that the gel didn't just improve intercourse, it made users and their partners obsessed with sex. Describing his partner, a man commented, "She just has this craving and she does not want me to stop." A participant noted simply, "Since I started using it, my partner is addicted to sex." These effects resulted in activities surrounding gel use becoming eroticized. A few couples described inserting the gel together as a critical and sensual part of foreplay; others stated that even having a conversation about the gel would cause arousal. Dikeledi commented, "When we talk about the gel we end up having sex because our minds just go there because he also likes the gel." Given the dramatic changes that the gel precipitated, community members occasionally speculated as to its contents. Thandi said, "I think there is something that they have put into the gel that they are not telling us about . . . because it makes sex so fun, actually." Zinzi recalled that at first she thought the gel was nothing more than a potential HIV prophylaxis, but after her libido improved dramatically she realized it was actually a sexual medication. Although participants were well aware that the trial was testing a microbicide designed to prevent HIV, their experiences suggested it was much more. For many, the gel was transformed from an experimental pharmaceutical into an aphrodisiac.

## SHIFTING PERCEPTIONS

Narratives of frequent and pleasurable sex permeated the community as participants and their partners shared their experiences with family, friends, and neighbors. As the gel became known as an aphrodisiac, women began enrolling for the primary purpose of improving their sex lives. A participant commented, "The thing that made me join the study is the gels because my neighbor told me that these gels make you have sex all the time. Then I told myself that I must go and get these gels so I can enjoy sex more." Women who were experiencing sexual difficulties were particularly eager. Zodwa reported:

> Sex was not my thing, and my partner was always wondering what was wrong with me for having no interest in sex but since I heard about the gel and what it is capable of, I could not wait to start using it. People were bragging about it, saying they are enjoying sex. I asked one of the women to give me one but she refused, saying I should wait until I qualified. She used to tell me that her partner always wants more sex and it did not bore her. Then I received mine and we tried it with my partner, and believe you me, we can never have sex without it. Sex was so enjoyable. My body started responding ardently to sex. . . . I was surprised because normally I'm not someone who likes sex.

Men also spoke to one another about the effects of the gel. A participant's partner recounted sharing his experience with the gel to a male friend, whom he then urged to have his girlfriend enroll in the trial because "when she uses the gel she wants more sex and she does not want you to stop." A number of men asked their partners to join the study in hopes that it would improve their sex lives. Men without regular partners sought to access the gel by purposely courting women on the trial. We were told of one man who refused to have sex with any woman not participating in the MDP301.

The gel's effect on sex played a role in how and when it was used. Those women who asserted that the gel was an aphrodisiac reported strong compliance. They did not forget to insert the gel prior to intercourse and were sure to go to the clinic to get more gels if their supply was diminishing.

As women sought to use the gel during every sexual encounter, so too did their partners. Wanting their sex to be as arousing as possible, male partners, including Kagiso's and Nomsa's, encouraged women always to insert the gel prior to sex. Kagiso commented, "He does not forget it. When we need to have sex he would ask me, 'Where are the gels?' . . . He always reminds me to use it." Nqobile had a similar experience: "I used it all the time and he would insert it for me sometimes. I was putting it under the pillow and inserted gel for every round." Like Nqobile and her partner, couples were also careful to ensure that gels were at hand whenever they engaged in sex. One participant's partner insisted that she store the gels at his residence so that they would always be available when she visited him.

Increased sexual pleasure motivated participants and their partners to modify earlier beliefs. Certain side effects, especially those associated with wetness, quickly became viewed as inconsequential by women when compared to the benefits of gel use. In an early interview, a participant stated that the gel caused noise during intercourse and that this would deter her from future use. But in a subsequent interview, she remarked that this had been only an initial impression. After realizing how good the gel made her feel, the noise no longer discouraged its utilization. Men who had previously complained that the gel could or did produce excessive wetness in their partners revised these views. Tebogo noted the gel made his partner so wet that the first round of sex felt like the second. Although he did not reveal his opinion to her, he told interviewers that he could not help but associate this wetness with cheating. As time progressed he realized that the gel made penetration significantly easier, especially when there was less time for foreplay. After witnessing the effects that this had on his partner's emotional state, Tebogo reconsidered his earlier views. He commented:

> I feel okay because she enjoys using the gel and I enjoy sex with her. Both of us enjoy sex together and she does not feel pain anymore. We enjoyed sex and I removed the mentality that I had that the gel made her too wet. . . . What I need is that she gets happiness and that also makes me happy. I don't want her to scream during sex because she feels pain. She must scream because she is enjoying it.

Tumelo's partner had similar reactions to the wetness caused by the gel. When Tumelo disclosed her participation in the trial, her partner accused her of having intercourse with another man. Once he realized that sex with the gel was significantly more pleasurable, his accusations ceased. Not only does he not question her fidelity, "now he reminds me to insert the gel because he said it is so nice when we have sex." In these instances, the assumed link between the gel, wetness, and promiscuity was abandoned.

Positive sexual experiences also altered men's attitudes regarding the toxicity of the gel and its potential for harm. In the previous chapter, we discussed Thaba's friend, who had asserted that the gel contained white witchcraft intended to kill the people of Orange Farm and Soweto. Thaba had also worried about the harm that the gel could potentially cause him, but this changed. He remarked, "She used it [the gel] for the whole month without telling me, but within two weeks of using it I noticed that there was something different about the way I was performing sexually. When I thought about black people being too African [uncivilized and resistant to change], I realized we are closing opportunities on many things and when we finally wake up it is too late because prevention is better than cure." Thaba revised his views as a result of his improved sexual encounters. The gel was transformed from a deadly pharmaceutical into a valuable tool for HIV prevention. Furthermore, beliefs regarding witchcraft were cast as backward and superstitious. Committed to make gel use a regular and accepted part of his sexual life, Thaba encouraged his partner to insert it in front of him despite her initial embarrassment. Like Thaba, Lindiwe's partner expressed concern that the gel was dangerous and could cause them both to fall ill. Anticipating that her partner would immediately notice an improvement in her performance and enjoyment, Lindiwe disclosed her trial participation prior to their initial gel use. After hesitantly agreeing to try the gel, he quickly discovered what Lindiwe had expected: sex was much better. She noted that he now portrays the trial as a positive endeavor that aids the community.

As couples praised the effects of the gel, they were conscious that their involvement in the trial was temporary. A participant asked, "What am I going to do if the medicine is no longer available? We are not going to enjoy sex the way we enjoyed it when I inserted the medicine." For those approaching the end of their enrollment, this issue became more acute. Phumla's partner asked if the gels would still be available after the enrollment period ended because "the gel persuades him to have sex more because sex is more enjoyable." When another participant informed her partner that she would not be able to use the gel after leaving the trial, "He was shocked that the time had come already for me to stop using the gel. I used to remind him that I would stop participating in the study eventually and I was only going to be using the gel for a year. He was shocked because our sex life had improved a lot with the gel. He would never hear me complain during sex like I used to before." The interviewer suggested that she could perhaps replicate the experience with a lubricant, such as K-Y, but the participant had never heard of such products and immediately inquired about their cost. She was worried that even if a lubricant provided a similar experience, she would be unable to afford it. Goitsemedime was also told that lubricant would alleviate the pain of intercourse but she was extremely reluctant to use another product: "I am not sure about that gel [lubricant] because I do not know if it is safe. The one I was using in the study was better because it was tested before and used it without having any problem. I am feeling bad that I will no longer use this gel and I do not like the one she told me about. I need this one and many people like it." Some women thus suggested that the trial should continue indefinitely. Zodwa proposed, "Maybe you should continue with this study so that we continue getting the gels." Puleng echoed this view: "Even if the study ends they should do something so that we continue getting the gel after 52 weeks because our partners will run away from us once they notice the changes because we will go back to how we were before we used gels." While improved sex was an important consequence of trial enrollment, Puleng's statement hints at another major outcome: improved relationships. Sex was not simply an exercise in enjoyment, but a tool for building a long-term love relationship.

## "IT MAKES YOUR LOVE GROW"

A fundamentally social act, sex creates and shapes relationships. As the trial progressed, it became apparent that the participants' sexual experiences had a profound impact on their sociality not only as partners but also as women. This newfound sociality was fashioned in part through women's experiences of speaking with one another while at the trial clinics. Each month, participants came to the clinics to report gel use, have their physical well-being checked, and participate in interviews. Throughout the duration of their enrollment, women were given appointments on the same day of every month. Because of the large number of women in the trial, the designated clinics dealt exclusively with MDP301 participants, but the limitations of space and staff resulted in long waits. On some days, women sat in the waiting room for up to eight hours before being seen by a nurse. Although these long delays initially annoyed some women, many eventually acknowledged that the clinic visits allowed them to forge new and unexpected bonds with their fellow participants. Encouraging her neighbor from Freedom Park to enroll, Mandisa commented that the female fellowship was more valuable than remuneration:

> I was telling this other girl to come here because she is sitting at home and not working. I told her to come so that she can be tested and know her own status. It is not about the money that you will get there, you will get friends, you will be part of a big family if you enroll in that study, you will whenever you have a problem [have someone] to talk to and all that. I even told her that when you start you will be thinking of the R150 but once you are inside you will lose interest in the R150 because of the other benefits that you will be getting.

As the same group of women gathered at the clinic each month, participants began striking up conversations with one another. Confident that everyone waiting to see the medical staff was enrolled, women openly shared their opinions of the gel. Given that the gel was used during intercourse, these conversations quickly turned to intimate subjects.

While sexual topics were usually discussed only between women who were close friends, the circumstances of the trial—a new pharmaceutical, long waits, and familiar faces—encouraged women to disregard this norm. Walking into the waiting room, one could overhear a number of explicit conversations. Women chatted about vaginal wetness and dryness, the frequency with which they engaged in sex, the sexual positions they and their partners preferred, their ability to orgasm more frequently while using the gel, and the responses of their partners to gel sex. During a focus group, participants described the content of waiting-room conversations:

**Respondent 1**: Most times we were talking about our partners and their reactions toward the gel. How did they feel when we inserted the gel and didn't insert it? Did they feel the same with or without the gel during sex? We were discussing those kinds of things.

***Respondent 2***: We were discussing that when you have inserted the gel your partner becomes free and happy and you become a youngster, especially for me as an older mother. I could feel that I was revived because he was no longer going out. We were coaching each other by saying let us treat our husbands well. My partner used to remind me to use the gel and I could feel that it was draining something from my private part so I was saying that it means I became a youngster. We were discussing those things, that the gel was working for us.

Reinforcing the perception that the gel was an aphrodisiac, these exchanges encouraged use. Girlie noted:

I was not dumping it [the gel]. I was just leaving it there, not using it, and when my clinic appointment for Week 4 neared I tried it and found that there is a difference in my sex life and I liked it. So coming here at the clinic helps because we talk about other people's fears and that helps them to overcome those fears and use the gel and now most of them are using the gel. They even say that their partners remind them of clinic visits when they see that the gel is finishing. We share a lot of experiences as women about the gel and once someone says something about it, you find that most women agree with that, so it is really helping people. Even if someone is quiet among the women and has doubts about the gel or has been dumping it, when she reaches home she will try it and then next month you will hear new stories from them about the gel.

While women appeared to be utilizing the gel as a result of these conversations, much more was occurring. Interactions in the waiting room allowed women to share knowledge and experiences in a way not previously available to them. Participants remarked that prior to joining the trial, they had never discussed such topics so openly with other women. Interestingly, these conversations continued even when men entered the clinics. Shocked that women would talk about sexual issues, one man reported fleeing the waiting area in embarrassment while others avoided entering the trial clinics altogether.

While ostensibly comparing experiences with the gel, participants in the waiting room also focused on the maintenance of sexual relationships. Lefu commented, "There are older people who tell us how to take care of a man when you are in the bedroom. Things like when you are angry and you do not want to have sex with your partner. Then older women say when you are angry do not say no when your man wants to have sex with you because you were not fighting about sex." Through talk of sexual fulfillment, women discussed love, commitment, and methods to sustain long-term relationships. Participants could share their insecurities and quandaries while receiving support and advice. If one woman had a problem, another offered a solution. In the focus group mentioned above, a third respondent added, "Some were discussing the problems they come across at home and how their partners were treating them. We were not necessarily talking about the gel only. If a person was stressed from home, we were able to talk about that to somebody who doesn't know you and give advice on how to handle the problem."

As bonds developed between women, phone numbers were exchanged and participants vowed to stay in contact during the intervening weeks between appointments. Lefu added, "Most of the time when you meet at the clinic you find that we socialize. Then we give each other our phone numbers and then start to visit each other. . . . We share problems and then we end up guiding each other. . . . I also share my problems with [a fellow participant] and that helps me." The clinic waiting room became a forum of validation and assistance, leading participants to anticipate their monthly appointments eagerly. Girlie remarked, "[Women] say they have problems but when they come to the clinic for those hours they forget them. They even wish it was a daily clinic, not because they came for money. . . . It turns out that the clinic does not only deal with gels and vaginas but with emotional issues indirectly. This clinic is really helping people with many things." Repudiating assertions that participation was motivated by financial gain, Girlie's statement illustrates the important role the trial played in shaping social relationships beyond the walls of the clinic.

One of the "many things" that the clinic and gel facilitated was love relationships between women and their partners. While the advice of other women was a factor in reshaping gender relationships, so was the newfound enjoyment of sex. Many participants stated that prior to joining the MDP301, they had sought to limit intimate contact because the discomfort associated with sex. This took not just a physical toll on their relationships but also an emotional one. Women claimed that sex was exhausting, causing them to be frustrated and argumentative. Couples experienced difficulty communicating and their time together could be fraught with disagreements and quarrels. Frequent fights reduced occasions for intimacy further, leading some men to avoid their homes and partners while potentially engaging in affairs. When this occurred, women felt insecure and worried about contracting sexually transmitted infections from unfaithful partners. These fears further motivated them to limit sexual contact with their men. Participants reported being able to break this vicious cycle of resentment and suspicion only after joining the trial. Commenting on the impact of gel use on her domestic life, a participant noted, "It has rebuilt my home, really, because we were always fighting when it comes to sex. I would tell my partner that I'm tired, just coming up with all kinds of excuses to avoid sex, but now that I'm using the gel I am very willing to have sex. All the tiredness I was complaining about has gone."

A number of women and men similarly noted that the ability to enjoy sex and engage in it more frequently profoundly altered partnered relationships and strengthened emotional bonds. Able to satisfy their partners sexually, men felt masculine and potent. Pretty noted, "When I orgasm he becomes happy because it means that he has become strong." As sex with their partners improved, men were more likely to visit their partners regularly and stay for longer periods. Kagiso explained, "It is a good relationship and we have been together for 14 years now. In the past he used not to come home but now since I started using the gel that has never happened. Maybe it is because he feels satisfied with me sexually." Dikeledi echoed these ideas: "It [the gel] makes me want sex every day because it makes him forget many things and when he is at work he forgets his friends and after work he comes straight home." A number of couples reported that better sex resulted in the partners spending greater amounts of time with each other. Not only were women's fears of male infidelity eased, communication was improved. Wanting to experience as much enjoyment as possible, participants began openly discussing how and when they achieved arousal. Several couples, including Zanele and her partner, noted that they had never engaged in explicit conversations of this nature prior to her trial enrollment. However, once these topics were broached, partners relished the ability to communicate frankly. Discussions regarding sex quickly led to conversations focusing on other aspects of their lives together. As communication increased, couples felt happier and more secure in their relationships.

As participants shared their experiences and desires with their partners at home and with other women in the waiting room, they reported becoming more self-confident. Continuing to engage in sexually explicit waiting-room conversations despite the presence of men was one way in which women publicly proclaimed their newfound power. In private, women also began asserting themselves rather than routinely deferring to convention or the desires of their partners. Sex was a primary tool through which women exercised their agency. A participant said, "Initially, I used to lack the confidence to initiate sex. But since I joined the study, I can just walk up to him and initiate something myself. There are a lot of things we learn in the study and you get to hear how other women do things." The encouragement of fellow participants motivated women to manage their own sexual relationships more actively. Many participants explicitly linked improved sex and agency. Phumla commented, "Sex is more enjoyable and I am more powerful and it is different from the time I was not using the gel." This newfound self-assurance was also evident outside their sexual relationships. Several women noted that they had confidence not just with their partner but with other men as well. For the first time, participants felt they could speak freely with men and were not hesitant about expressing their opinions.

Many participants noticed that their partners were increasingly attentive and affectionate. Mosa reported that not only was her partner more energetic, he regularly called her "hot," which Mosa found extremely flattering. She added, "He was not the same as before I started using the gel. Now he started saying many things and he promised me a lot of things. Like, he promised to buy me a cell phone." Many others also described being flattered and spoiled by their men for the first time. Through compliments and gifts, men were showing affection in tangible ways. Women viewed these gestures as proof of their partners' commitment and devotion. As a result, many participants credited the gel with a primary role in linking sex to love. A participant commented, "I think when you use the gel it makes your love grow because there are no complaints like my partner asking me why today do you feel wet. I am saying this because when you are with your partner he feels like having sex with you all the time." She added, "The gel treats me well." Echoing these sentiments, Lindiwe described the changes in her relationship: "I feel as though I am a queen. . . . He is treating me very well, unlike before. Before I started using the gel, we would fight a lot because I used to get dry when having sex. . . . Now he is coming to see me almost every day. He tells me that he loves me and things like that." It is noteworthy that both of these statements invoke notions of wet and dry. Building on and modifying narratives linking ideal vaginal state to male devotion, the gel became a tool that enabled women to hold onto their men and to secure their love through sexual experience. Once their sociality within a relationship was guaranteed, other aspects of the women's existence were subsequently enhanced. A participant said simply, "Everything in my life has improved."

While researchers have asserted that dry sex is a means through which norms and expectations are expressed, we believe that it is important to acknowledge the ways these ideals are experienced. As researchers sought to identify an innovative way to prevent HIV, women in the trial found a different but similarly revolutionary use for a new pharmaceutical. Drawing from long-standing assumptions regarding a bodily locus of femininity centered on the vagina, the gel was credited with transforming women's bodies, turning discomfort into pleasure. A meaningful vehicle for conceptualizing relationships, sex tangibly built sociality through enactment. Providing men with sexual experiences that other women could not, participants reconfigured their relationships with intimate partners while forging bonds with one another. Most importantly, these transformations were precipitated by women's physical pleasure. Desire and arousal fundamentally altered women's perceptions of themselves, emboldening them to assert their sexual capital.

# Experiencing
# Efficacy

Although researchers continue to invest in microbicide development, any new product will be released to the public only after the conclusion of a successful phase III trial. Through careful data collection and statistical methods, researchers seek to transform the hope of microbicides into the reality of HIV prevention. For doctors, researchers, and microbicide advocates, this entails proving efficacy under the "perfect conditions" of a clinical trial. To determine the effectiveness of PRO 2000/5, the MDP301 adhered to established protocols. Participants were randomized to one of three gels—a placebo, a gel containing 0.5 percent PRO 2000/5, or a gel containing 2 percent PRO 2000/5—and the drug was assessed by comparing these different arms. Efficacy is most often determined through an intent-to-treat analysis, which includes all participants, even if they missed doses or failed to complete the trial (Heise et al. 2011). These calculations are completed at research institutions in the Global North, far away from where the trials are conducted. After the conclusion of the MDP301, trial data, coupled with the results of medical tests and seroconversion rates, was collated in the United Kingdom. In most cases, the results of a trial are announced only after extensive data cleaning and analysis has been conducted, usually many months after the last participant has left the trial.

As medical researchers in the MDP301 gathered information, participants were equally curious to know if the gel "worked." Women had their own benchmarks, which differed significantly from those of trial staff. Whereas the MDP301 focused on quantitative indicators, women concentrated on the immediate embodied experience of gel use. Concerned about the gel's effect on their bodies, participants and their partners took an active role in evaluating the physical changes they were experiencing after joining the trial. While women reported feeling a number of sensations while using the gel, the most noticeable immediate effect of gel use was increased vaginal discharge, particularly after engaging in intercourse.[1] Drawing from beliefs regarding the ubiquity of dirt and the use of liquids to purify bodies, women—including Zanele, Nomsa, Andiswa, Zinzi, Goitsemedime, Kagiso, and Boikanyo—asserted that this discharge was evidence that the gel was cleansing the vagina. The gel's ability to remove impurities led these women to claim that it had alleviated a number of complaints, including vaginal itching, vaginal sores, rashes, menstrual pains, and abdominal pains, as well as protecting them from HIV infection. Consequently, many women enrolled in the trial said that they did not need to wait for statisticians in the United Kingdom to review the trial data; they knew that the gel was efficacious.

The cleansing and reinvigorating characteristics that many women attributed to the gel are noted in acceptability studies of microbicides (Bass 2002; Mantell, Morar, et al. 2006). However, these narratives are usually explained as arising from "misperceptions" of the gel. In clinical trials such as the MDP301, clinic staff placed emphasis on imparting the "correct" knowledge to trial participants regarding the unproven effects of the gel and the efficacy of condoms, but these messages were often unable to alter persistent beliefs. Participants evaluated microbicides not by uncritically accepting biomedical meaning but by integrating everyday experiences of gel use into existing beliefs regarding the body. Through their substantiveness, pharmaceuticals acquire meaning within a local context (van der Geest and Whyte 1989; Whyte et al. 2002). This was particularly true of the gel, which produced significant bodily responses. Applying their own criteria for efficacy, community residents actively reconfigured relationships between themselves and medical researchers. Emphasizing their own gold standard, participants claimed power and agency within the research process.

## CONDOMS AND BLOCKAGE

While microbicides were being hailed as a potential method of halting the spread of HIV, a proven efficacious alternative already existed: condoms. Reflecting the frustration of many South Africans, an MDP301 participant commented, "we have access to condoms but still we have many people who are HIV positive." Although condoms are able to prevent HIV transmission, the AIDS epidemic in sub-Saharan Africa has yet to be reversed, in part because condoms have not been used consistently or reliably (Hearst and Chen 2004; Wojcicki and Malala 2001). Underlying this problem is the difficulty that women experience in convincing their male partners to use condoms. In addition, the possibility of obtaining cash or gifts motivates women to engage in condom-free sex (Hunter 2002; Kaufman and Stavrou 2002; Leclerc-Madlala 2003; Wojcicki and Malala 2001). Furthermore, women's concerns about HIV infection may be secondary to the risk of spoiling romantic relationships by insisting on condom use (Sobo 1995). Condoms are often worn only in risky, temporary sexual encounters, and are considered antithetical to long-term intimate relationships based on mutual trust and respect, such as marriage (Chimbiri 2007; MacPhail and Campbell 2001). These views were inculcated in part through early public health campaigns that stressed the association between condoms and risky relationships (Sobo 1995). Seeking general explanations for unevenness in condom use, researchers tend to focus on gender inequalities and patriarchal dominance in South African society (Thege 2009). However, the situation is much more complicated. While condoms function as effective receptacles to contain semen and limit HIV risk, they are not always conceptualized solely in terms of their instrumentality. The condom is a sign-vehicle that conveys multiple, often contradictory, meanings that shape use and nonuse in several ways (Middelthon 2001).

Expressing the views of many Sowetans and Orange Farmers, one participant said that condoms are utilized "once in a while" and this occurs only when the male partner "feels like using it." Women often blamed men for discouraging or, in most cases, forbidding the use of condoms. While male agency played a role in the use or nonuse of condoms, so did perceptions of the relationship itself. As a male Sowetan succinctly noted, "I use a condom when having sex with someone I do not trust." Elaborating on this statement, another male said that condom use was important only in newly established relationships: "For the first three months I will use condoms and then leave it later on." Long-term partners are trusted to be faithful, leading many to assert that condoms are more appropriate with one-night stands. A married man said, "If it's my wife we won't use it [condom], because you trust her, she's the lady of the house. But these other ones outside, you can also throw on a plastic bag for extra protection, because if it's somebody from outside, you can never know with them." Given the association of condoms with affairs, asking a partner to use a condom could result in accusations of infidelity. When a woman attempts to introduce condoms into a long-term relationship, one man said, "What goes through the mind of a man is that you are starting to cheat. It means you have been cheating all along and now you want me to use this thing." Consequently, a reluctance to insist on condom use was intimately tied not just to the sexual but also the social relationships between partners.

In addition to negotiating the social repercussions of condom use, women and men were conscious of using a technology that could potentially fail or cause physical discomfort. We were told numerous stories of condoms either coming off or rupturing during sex. A woman who also believed that pubic hairs made holes in condoms noted that "you can put on a condom the right way, but when you are very busy, bah! [the condom bursts]." While a burst condom was acknowledged to be ineffective in preventing HIV transmission, it was also thought to endanger an individual's health in other ways. Women reported condoms becoming lodged in their vaginas, sometimes for an extended period. A participant commented, "You will be surprised when you pass urine to see a condom coming out." It was believed that whether condoms slid off or burst, latex left in the womb could potentially block the vagina and cause a buildup of fluids, which would precipitate a number of health problems.

Even correctly functioning condoms were thought to pose a health risk. Some people suspected that condoms were contaminated with diseases. This was occasionally expressed in terms of a popular South African conspiracy theory that cast condoms as containers of diseases designed to exterminate black people. Some alluded to the contamination of condoms with HIV or alleged that they contained microscopic organisms or virus-like "worms." As discussed in the third chapter, these rumors reflect larger discussions about racial relationships and spiritual insecurities. These narratives existed alongside others linking the everyday experiences of using condoms to beliefs about the body. When utilizing condoms, a number of people reported having genital rashes, vaginal dryness, and pain during sex prompting concerns over their safety. While men noted that condoms caused skin irritation, women worried that condom lubricants accumulated in the womb and caused infections. A female Orange Farmer said, "I used to have a rash inside my vagina and I would feel pain and get swollen on the sides." Thaba summed up the objections of many when he commented, "Yes, they are able to prevent HIV but they have a lot of complications: They burst, the lubricant is not enough, and I experience pain in my kidneys after using condoms, so I think it fills me with a lot of air in my stomach." Thaba noted that after using condoms he often felt lower abdominal pain and general discomfort. Although condoms were generally believed to be efficacious in preventing HIV, they were also viewed as unreliable and potentially dangerous to one's health.

While some individuals no doubt experienced allergies and other reactions to latex, these anti-condom sentiments were amplified by beliefs regarding the flow of bodily fluids during intercourse. Procreative sex is portrayed as the intermingling of a man's white blood (semen) and a woman's red blood. Conceptualized as an exchange of gifts, fluid transfer is essential for reproduction and for the constitution of personhood (Thornton 2008). The movement of red and white blood is critical not only for fertility, but also in terms of individual development. Signifying internal processes as well as social relatedness, fluids mark the ways in which bodies interact with the world and others (Grosz 1994; Kristeva 1982). Consequently, failing to release blood through sexual intercourse or blocking the free flow of seminal and vaginal fluids between partners results in negative health outcomes and the erosion of personhood (Niehaus 2002; Taylor 1990). Among adolescents in the South African lowveld, facial acne, irritability, and dark patches of skin are believed to be results of insufficient sexual contact (Collins and Stadler 2000). Girls reported symptoms of "abdominal discomfort, bodily swelling, headaches (the blood was 'blocked in the head'), tiredness, sores on the body, infections, weight gain and skin changes," and temporary infertility because of hormonal contraception that caused sporadic spotting and low volumes of menstrual fluid (Wood and Jewkes 2006:112). These notions are embedded in the idea of the fractal person (Taylor 1990) or the "dividual" (Niehaus 2002), which unlike the bounded individual is constructed through the reciprocal exchange of fluids. From this perspective, sex with a condom is not really sex at all (Collins and Stadler 2000).

Given these beliefs, condoms can be implicated in obstructing the flow of substances within and between bodies, resulting in illness (Thornton 2008). Anxieties about condoms causing blockage are relatively widespread, particularly in long-term relationships, where the sharing and exchange of fluids is most desirable (Allen and Heald 2004; Gupta and Weiss 1993; Sobo 1993; Taylor 1990). Thaba's earlier statement—that condoms fill his stomach with air and make him ill—references his body's inability to absorb a woman's blood during intercourse. While several of the men we interviewed expressed similar opinions, some took steps to alleviate their apprehension by rendering the condom permeable on purpose. Men in one focus group admitted to puncturing holes in condoms to make "sex taste sweeter," expressing a desire for the mixing of semen and vaginal fluids. Reflecting a concern held by several men, that their bodily fluids not be wasted, a younger man refrained from condom use because he did not want his semen to "end up in the dustbin." Another asserted that using condoms meant that his future progeny "would be killed." The condom stood in direct opposition to fluid flow, creating blockage and therefore causing ill health. Consequently, narratives of illness-causing condoms can be correlated with core beliefs about maintaining and controlling the flow of sexual fluids. In contrast to condoms, the gel was regarded as a technology that encouraged flow. Thaba's negative reactions to the condom were absent when Precious used the gel, which he viewed as a preferable alternative. Unlike latex, the gel permitted the comingling of fluids.

## DIRT, CLEANLINESS, AND FLOW

A critical aspect of procreative sex, the flow of bodily fluids also ensures personal cleanliness and protection from harmful pollutants. Transcending bounded bodies, beliefs regarding pollution act as a fundamental framework from which the social world can be explained. Mary Douglas (1966) describes pollution as contextually situated matter out of place, which disrupts or blurs classificatory models. As such, dirt is destabilizing. Bodily orifices and their secretions are situated at the margins where the self meets the world. Douglas writes, "We cannot possibly interpret ritual concerning excreta, breast milk, saliva and the rest unless we are prepared to see in the body a symbol of society, and to see the power and danger credited to social structure reproduces in small on the human body" (115). Douglas's remarks are particularly relevant for understanding participants' attitudes toward microbicide gels, which are inserted into and then flow out of reproductive cavities. Incorporated into southern African ontologies of pollution, microbicides are once again transformed into a technology of signification.

In South Africa, attitudes and actions focusing on dirt are intrinsically linked to the body and structure everyday practices. Shaped by a variety of factors, including tradition (Green 1999; Hammond-Tooke 1989; Ngubane 1977), Christian missionary teaching (Comaroff 1985; Comaroff and

Comaroff 1997; Moffat 1842), biomedical notions (Department of Health 1997; Manganyi 1974), and marketing (Burke 1996), these beliefs are ubiquitous and undergird conceptions of the self and well-being (Ashforth 2005:156). A common theme in health narratives, the transfer of dirt-removing liquids through bodies is part of a regular cleansing regime to maintain good health and prevent illness (Thornton 2008). Biological processes such as digestion, urination, and defecation naturally cleanse the body, but individuals also take steps to flush pollutants using other means. To ensure abdominal health, adults regularly administer enemas to themselves and their children (Lusu et al. 2001; Moore and Moore 1998). One survey conducted in KwaZulu-Natal reported that 89 percent of the 107 infants surveyed received enemas, often more than once a week within the first 3 months of life. The most common reasons given were constipation and the need to be "cleaned out" by visibly removing contaminants (Bland et al. 2004). To accomplish this task, solutions of salt, herbal mixes, topical antiseptics, or soap were most commonly used, although more caustic agents such as bleach, vinegar, potassium dichromate, copper sulphate, and potassium permanganate have also been documented (Ashforth 2005; Dunn et al. 1991; Segal and Tim 1979). This varied list reflects a long-standing trend whereby individuals test and incorporate new products into existing hygiene patterns, such as using petroleum jelly or body lotion to reinvent the southern African practice of "smearing," rubbing fat on the body to enhance beauty or health (Burke 1996:171).

Like the digestive tract, the vagina is considered to be a conduit for pollution into and out of the body. The women of Soweto and Orange Farm often spoke of their vaginas as reservoirs within which dirt collected.[2] An important natural cleansing mechanism analogous to digestion, menstruation removes dirt via the flow of blood (Jewkes and Wood 1999; Leclerc-Madlala 2002). Consequently, menstrual blood is widely considered to be a source of potential pollution and illness (De Heusch 1980; Hammond-Tooke 1981; Ngubane 1976; Niehaus 2002; Pauw 1990). Trial participants regularly stated avoiding sexual intercourse when menstruating for fear that the dirt being expelled would cause their partner to become ill. Zanele remarked, "You are dirty and you expel the dirt and give it to your partner. When you menstruate you are cleaning inside your womb and you are giving your partner your dirt." Describing his reluctance to engage in intercourse with a menstruating woman, a man commented, "I am scared because it is dirty blood and moreover, it is easy for a woman to become pregnant if you have sex with her when she is menstruating." For many, menstruation and fertility were immediately linked. An absence of dirt is not only necessary for health, but also for conception. Through the natural cleaning process of menstruation, the vagina is made ready for pregnancy (Leclerc-Madlala 2002).

While women relied on menstruation as a natural purgative process, they also engaged in a number of regimens to cleanse their vaginas. Some participants recalled that their female elders instructed them to clean the outside as well as the inside of their vaginas by using their fingers, to remove "dirty stuff." Reflecting the concerns and habits of many women, a participant described her own cleansing habits as follows:

> I wash it [external genitalia] with my hand and I insert the finger inside to remove all the discharge because this smells bad. So, you have to remove this all the time, because if you only wash over it, it is not enough. I mean you cannot use a scrubbing brush or anything when you are washing. You have to insert the finger and remove all the dirt because if you do not do that, the dirt will come out while you are walking and get trapped in your underwear and it will start smelling. Yes, when you are washing you have to remove it [dirt].

As the participant notes, the vagina cannot be scoured with an abrasive device, leading many women to rely not just on their fingers but also on the specialized properties of cleansing agents to do this work. Building on earlier missionary ideas of bodily discipline and cleanliness, soaps such as Sunlight have been popular throughout southern Africa for decades (Burke 1996). The result of marketing messages and personal experimentation, douching with a wide range of substances, including bar or laundry soap, antiseptics, vinegar, salt water, industrial detergents, and to a lesser extent, local preparations from plant or animal materials, was a common and routine practice for trial participants and women throughout South Africa (Morar and Karim 1998; Myer et al. 2006; Scorgie et al. 2009).[3]

In a result unanticipated by the trial coordinators, the gel became another product that was incorporated into vaginal cleansing narratives and practices. Similar to douching and enemas, the gel was thought to cleanse the body through the flow of liquids. Many women reported that the most noticeable effect of gel use was vaginal discharge. Furthermore, discharge resulting from gel use was often perceived to have a different color, texture, or smell from everyday vaginal secretions. During a focus group a participant asked the moderator, "I want to know why before you insert the gel it [vaginal discharge] is yellow but after sex it becomes white." Before the moderator could respond, another participant interjected, "I am answering her question. It's because after having sex it cleans you. That is why it changes color and becomes white." This assertion was echoed by many women—including Zanele, Nomsa, Andiswa, Zinzi, Phumla, Goitsemedime, Busi, Kagiso, and Boikanyo—who claimed that vaginal discharge was evidence that dirt was "drawn out," "dragged," and "flushed" from the vagina by the gel. Andiswa said, "I think it cleans. Sometimes you have impurities inside but you are not aware of them." She, like others, came to this conclusion after witnessing polluting substances being expelled. Boikanyo noted, "I also believe that since I started using the gel, my vagina is clean. [The gel] comes out with all the dirty things that should not be there." Participants reported that over time, discharge tended to become clear and odorless, which was interpreted as a sign of vaginal cleanliness and further proof of the gel's effectiveness.

While vaginal discharge provided strong evidence that the gel was removing impurities, the chemical potency of PRO 2000/5 was marshaled as further proof. Participants were aware that they had been randomized to one of three trial arms: a gel containing 2 percent PRO 2000/5, 0.5 percent PRO 2000/5, and a placebo. Despite the trial being double-blinded, women believed that they could identify which gel they were using based on the side effects it produced.[4] Those participants who did not notice symptoms or bodily changes often asserted that they were using an inactive gel: "But in my view I think maybe I had been using the placebo gel because I did not experience any side effects. When I started to use the gel I thought maybe I was going to develop a rash but I never experienced that."[5] In contrast, another participant stated, "I believe that I was given one with percentages [0.5 percent or 2 percent] because of the way things happen in my body." Those participants who reported experiencing "side effects" were more likely to believe that they were using one of the active gels, those that contained PRO 2000/5. Goitsemedime knew immediately that the gel was acting in her body because "when I inserted the gel it felt as if I have applied medication on the wound and there was a tingling." The sensation and viscosity of the gel were often criteria for determining its potency: "If it was a placebo I think I could feel that. It feels something like water but in this [gel] I feel that there are some chemicals in my body that I have inserted."[6] A few participants sought to determine which gel they had received by "testing" it in various homemade experiments. One combined the gel with semen from a used condom, reporting that "the gel sunk down and the sperm rose up." Because the two substances appeared to remain separate, she concluded that the gel contained PRO 2000/5. Those women who believed they possessed an active gel—albeit one that had yet to be scientifically proven effective—stressed that PRO 2000/5 was affecting their bodies not only through side effects but also by its ability to cleanse.

Despite overwhelmingly agreement that the active gel was an effective cleaning agent, women disagreed about the potential results of this process. The most popularly debated issue was pregnancy. Prior to the introduction of the gel, HIV prevention was linked to pregnancy prevention, as condoms were employed for both tasks. Because the gel did not use a physical barrier, relying instead on a chemical compound, women disagreed over what, if any, effect it would have on reproduction. Some simply equated the gel with a condom and said that it also inhibited pregnancy. However, others employed ideas regarding the active chemicals in the gels containing PRO 2000/5 that also impacted attitudes regarding pregnancy: "The sperms are going to die before coming into contact with the chemical of the gel. But if it is the placebo, yes, you can become pregnant." Still others appealed to the logic of cleansing to guide their assessment, stating that the ability of the gel to flush pollutants from the vagina would ensure that sperm were expelled as well, thereby preventing pregnancy. A participant noted, "After inserting the gel it cleans me inside for three days and I think I am not going to be pregnant because it cleans everything. It all comes out." Another added, "I think it prevents it [pregnancy] because since I have been using the gel I can see the sperms coming out of the vagina and I think the gel protects my womb against the sperms entering the womb."

But this same pattern of reasoning, which prompted some women to assert that the gel's cleansing ability would prevent pregnancy, led many others to the opposite conclusion. Citing the importance of an unpolluted vagina for pregnancy, several participants said that gel use increased the likelihood of conception. Busi remarked, "I think the gel removes the dirt from the body and in that way it might be possible to fall pregnant while using the gel." These women emphasized that this was not mere conjecture;

it was clearly proven by the many participants who became pregnant while enrolled.[7] A participant noted, "Many people are getting pregnant, those who are not using the condom. . . . The gel is stronger that those contraceptives. They actually become pregnant. It opens up the tubes." This statement alludes to the ability of the gel to facilitate the flow of fluids through the body, thereby "opening" the fallopian tubes. The view that the gel was more potent than contraceptives was expressed by others. Zanele felt that the gel counteracted hormonal contraception because it "cleanses the injectable [hormonal] contraceptives out of the system." Zanele claimed to have firsthand knowledge of the gel's abilities: after failing to conceive for months, she became pregnant while using the gel. She said, "The gel is good for women because it has cleaned me and I fell pregnant." Zanele was not alone. Many others reported unsuccessfully attempting to become pregnant for months or years until joining the trial. One participant described being told by a private doctor that she would never have a child, only to become pregnant while on the trial. Overjoyed, she praised the gel for its ability to increase fertility.

These responses to the gel were unexpected by the MDP301 designers and coordinators. This is in part because microbicide safety and tolerability studies categorize vaginal discharge as an "adverse event" (Mayer et al. 2003), attributing it to expulsion of the gel and normal cervical discharge (Van Damme et al. 2000). Cast as a largely unremarkable side effect, vaginal discharge was viewed as discrete from the main purpose of PRO 2000/5: HIV prevention. However, side effects that health professionals might dismiss as proximally caused could be interpreted experientially by those using the drug as proof of efficacy (Etkin 1988; Etkin 1992). Nina Etkin (1992:102) writes, "That which may be defined as a side effect in terms of biomedical construction may be embraced as a pre-requisite part of the process that demonstrates healing." For some trial participants, vaginal discharge was not simply a side effect; it was evidence of PRO 2000/5's ability to encourage flow and rid the body of polluted substances. Like the use of Pond's body lotion for smearing or Dettol for enemas, PRO 2000/5 was incorporated into existing ideas regarding the body and cleanliness. The expulsion of fluid from the vagina became a primary rather than side effect of the gel. These perceptions are reflected in international acceptability studies: data collected during the phase I trial of PRO 2000/5 reveals that while American women frequently complained about "leakage" and viewed it as a deterrent to gel use, South African women did not (Morrow et al. 2003:661). For women in the MDP301, vaginal discharge powerfully proved that the gel was "doing something" positive within their bodies.

## PROTECTING WOMEN

Participants often stated that the ability of PRO 2000/5 to flush vaginal pollution resulted in significantly improved reproductive health. Although the women were well aware that PRO 2000/5 was still being tested, they claimed that the gel facilitated menstruation, cured vaginal infections, and prevented STIs. Menstrual difficulties were one of the many vaginal issues that PRO 2000/5 was thought to address. Participants claimed that the gel aided the body's natural processes during menstruation, reduced menstrual pain, and facilitated an optimal and reliable flow. Kagiso reported, "The gel has cleaned my body. For instance, last time when I was menstruating I noticed that dirty blood was coming out and I think it was accumulated in my body." Similarly, another participated noted, "Before I joined the study I used to have a problem with my period that it would flow very strong. But since I used the gel I do not have that problem." Other women claimed that after using the gel for a few months, their menstrual cycles became regular and predicable for the first time. One participant complained of previously experiencing vaginal bleeding at intermittent intervals throughout the month but stated that this had stopped after she began using the gel. PRO 2000/5 was also credited with resolving vaginal problems resulting from childbirth: "I gave birth last year. Then they did not remove everything in my womb. Then I have taken different medicines and nothing helped me until I used the gel. Today I am fine."

Many participants—including Zinzi, Andiswa, Goitsemedime, Nomsa, and Kagiso—also claimed that the gel effectively treated vaginal infections, which were commonly described in terms of a discolored or milky discharge, a strong unpleasant odor, and itching. As with menstrual problems, the cleansing abilities of PRO 2000/5 were credited. Andiswa was confident that she was being given an active gel:

> Before I started using the gel . . . I used to get a thick discharge with a foul smell. The gel has helped me with that problem because there is no smell anymore. I used to wash frequently because of that smell, but now

when I wake up I can just wash my hands, brush my teeth, and make myself a cup of coffee. I think it was the gel that helped me with the smell because it vanished after I started using the gel.[8]

Kagiso's discharge had been so heavy that she used "diapers" to catch the flow but she reported that the gel had completely alleviated this problem. For women who suffered from recurrent genital herpes, such as Boikanyo, the gel was also credited with easing and preventing outbreaks. These assertions were not confined to participants but echoed by partners and family members. Hendrick recalled that the gel had relieved his partner "of her discharge and many other problems that women experience. She says it treats her well and that's what has persuaded me to believe that it is a good gel." As more and more women credited PRO 2000/5 with curing infections, stories of the gel's healing abilities circulated around the community. Friends and relatives of women suffering from vaginal problems were encouraged to gain access to the gel. Lulama commented, "Before joining the study, I used to have vaginal thrush. My mother felt that the gel would help relieve the thrush and told me to try it. After using the gel for about two months, I no longer had a problem with vaginal thrush. I think the gel stopped it." Like claims of the gel increasing sexual pleasure, stories of the protective properties of PRO 2000/5 motivated some community members to enroll in the trial.

While participants stated that the gel alleviated infections and sought to have access to it, they were simultaneously prescribed topical creams and antibiotics as a routine part of the MDP301's treatment protocol. Participants, including Boikanyo, Goitsemedime, and Lulama, received medications from the trial clinic for their infections, but these treatments were seldom mentioned. During the infrequent cases when antibiotics were discussed, the gel was still ascribed the key role in the patient's recovery. A participant commented, "I had a problem of discharge but since I came to the study they gave me treatment and the gel and the problem has been resolved. I think the gel is doing something inside my body." Women did not doubt the efficacy of clinical treatment but regarded the cleansing properties of the gel as essential for the completion of the healing process. As a result, the gel was compared to and equated with vaginal medicines: "I take the gel as a vaginal cream because sometimes you find that I have a problem with discharge so when I go to the clinic they give me a vaginal cream so I can clean every dirty thing in my womb. So this gel is similar to a vaginal cream so my mind tells me that this gel is something that does not like dirty things." Although the gel was thought to cleanse the vagina, this was made possible through the presence of PRO 2000/5, a chemical compound. Consequently, the gel appeared to contain an active pharmacological agent similar in every respect to other medications. But unlike conventional treatments, which were not perceived to remove dirt, the gel's effectiveness was demonstrated through the presence of flow and discharge.

Participants were also inclined to stress the effectiveness of the gel over antibiotics because conventional treatment regimens administered prior to the trial had often failed to result in lasting recoveries. Goitsemedime described her experience as follows: "I was changing underwear every time. People told me to wash with different things but it couldn't help. I even consulted different clinics and they gave some tubes to use but it couldn't help either. Since I started using the gel the discharge is no longer there. The gel has helped me a lot." Like Goitsemedime, others who had previously suffered from vaginal infections regularly reported seeking care at local clinics. Although medication was utilized, these drugs were described as either granting only a temporary cessation of symptoms or being completely ineffective. For example, Themba recounted having a recurrent rash for several months that she feared was cancer. Despite receiving treatment from a local clinic for a six-month period, the rash persisted. It was only after Themba joined the trial and began using the gel that the rash disappeared. For many like her, lasting relief from reproductive health complaints was achieved only following enrollment in the MDP301.

But PRO 2000/5 was thought to do more than treat what were seen as spontaneous and chronic infections. Participants consistently claimed it could protect women from diseases contracted through sexual contact with men. Goitsemedime, Tshepiso, Kagiso, Precious, and many others all said that the active gel prevented HIV. As they described PRO 2000/5's power to protect women from STIs and HIV, the gel's ability to remove pollutants from the body was a significant and recurrent theme. Noting that he encouraged his partner to use the gel because it effectively cleaned her vagina and prevented infections, Hendrick stated, "I think what happens is when I come with a sickness and I transmit to her, then the gel automatically destroys that sickness on contact so that the sickness does not affect her." Kagiso commented, "I think it cleanses the body and nothing foreign will be left in the body. And I think it will help to prevent this HIV epidemic because it cleanses the body." Asked to explain her belief that PRO 2000/5 prevented HIV transmission, a participant said, "When it comes out it removes the dirt. That is why I say it must remove the virus as well." Witnessing the flow of semen and gel out of the body, participants claimed the efficacy of PRO 2000/5 was visibly demonstrated.

Statements stressing the role of cleansing in HIV prevention were supplemented by personal insights and science-like discourse. After noting that the gel flushed out pollutants, Busi spoke of her experience of the gel as well as its medicinal properties: "I think [the gel] can prevent HIV infection because when I have inserted it I feel it moving through my body and working. It smells like methylated spirits." When providing specific descriptions of how PRO 2000/5 medically and biologically "worked," many people said that it created a barrier inside a woman's body, blocking and killing sexually transmitted viruses while continuing to allow the exchange of fluids during intercourse. Andiswa said that the gel "turns into water and gets inside the tubes in a woman's body" and then "shuts the tubes." Often invoking physiology, several women described bodily sites on which PRO 2000/5 acted: "I think the gel can protect me because it covers the cervix. When the cervix is covered, sexually transmitted infections are not able to reach the cervix as it is a vulnerable place to infections." For others, the vagina was the locus of potential infection and protection. A male partner described this mechanism: "When a woman inserts the gel, it covers the walls of the vagina, and then when you penetrate, even when you release your sperm, it does not have that power to go in through the layers of the vagina. It does not have power and it does nothing." Also focusing on the vaginal walls, Tumelo said, "I think it [PRO 2000/5] is right [efficacious] because the gel makes walls strong; it is like building a stop-nonsense [a precast wall typical in townships]. It uses chemicals so it can become strong." As Tumelo indicated, the presence of an active pharmacological substance was seen as a critical component of the gel's effectiveness in preventing STIs.

Narratives asserting that PRO 2000/5 was effective in inhibiting reproductive diseases drew from widespread assumptions that linked dirt to biomedical illness categories. Several women, such as Zanele, attributed STIs to dirty blood or semen in the vagina, while others frequently fused notions of dirt, disease, and STIs. Stating a commonly held belief, a participant said, "Bacterium is dirt. And in my knowledge it means that it is the same as an STD." Throughout South Africa, STIs and HIV are regularly equated with pollution through their capacity to create bodily and social disorder (Henderson 2004). Like dirt, STIs have the ability to cause damage to physical bodies as well as to intimate reproductive relationships. If STIs are equated with pollution and the gel removes pollution, it was logical to assume, as many women did, that the gel could also prevent and cure STIs. As a participant noted, "Let's say my partner had 'dirt sickness' [STI] and I did not know about that but since I use the gel I would not need to go to the clinic or have a problem with STIs." In many of their statements, women conflated the cleansing, shielding, and antiviral properties of PRO 2000/5: "I thought that it was searching for diseases inside me while protecting me at the same time by removing all the dirt, even if I had come in contact with someone who is infected with HIV." Zinzi echoed these comments: "I had discharge before I started using it and I realized that it is a medicine that prevents sexually transmitted diseases. The way I see it, it is a powerful medicine because I have seen how it works." She added that the gel clearly prevented HIV because it "cleanses dirty blood that has a virus." Rather than separable processes, cleaning, curing, and protecting were all outcomes of a single mechanism. Flowing between the internal and external, the gel purified the body by removing transgressive substances. In contrast, antibiotics prescribed to treat vaginal infections were static and therefore seldom credited with precipitating lasting reproductive health. PRO 2000/5 was interpreted locally as experiences of vaginal discharge were placed within an existing epistemology of pollution.

As final evidence of PRO 2000/5's ability to protect women from STIs, participants pointed to their own HIV status. Despite rarely using condoms, women commented that they and others remained HIV negative throughout the trial. Zodwa remarked, "I think it [PRO 2000/5] is working. If it wasn't working at least some of us coming here would have tested HIV positive by now and not everyone who comes here uses condoms. Like myself, I don't use condoms at all, but we always test negative to HIV so that means the gel is working." After exiting the study, Kagiso, Precious, and Lebogang similarly invoked their continued status as HIV negative to confidently state that the gel was efficacious. Lebogang added, "I feel the gel working and now we are just waiting for the announcement that it is working." For other participants, the gel's abilities were demonstrated through crises. In one dramatic example, PRO 2000/5 was credited with not only preventing HIV but also removing all evidence of semen after a woman had suffered a sexual assault:

The gel is a hundred times better [than condoms] because last week my cousin saw the container of gel and she asked me about the gel after seeing it. Then when she went to a party, she stole two gels from me, without telling me. Then while she was still at the party, they raped her and when she came to Bara [Chris Hani Baragwanath Hospital] they checked her and they found that nothing had infected her. So, they asked her what she used before they raped her because they could not see any sperm in her womb. Then she told them that she stole the gels from me and used them.

Stories such as this underscored many of the predominant assumptions regarding the cleansing and protective properties of PRO 2000/5: even in the face of sexual assault, women who use the gel are shielded from HIV infection. However, none of the women interviewed stated that the PRO 2000/5 could cure HIV if it had been previously contracted.

These assertions caused consternation among trial coordinators for two reasons. First, it seemed as if the MDP301's key message—that PRO 2000/5 required systematic testing before its efficacy could be assessed—was not being understood. In fact, women were well aware that PRO 2000/5 was still in the process of being scientifically assessed. Phumla stated, "[The clinic staff] told me that they are still doing research to see if it prevents infections, but I think it prevents HIV and STIs because it has cleaned my urine, blood, and cured menstrual pain." Many participants were unable to resolve these differing perspectives easily. Expressing the dissonance between clinic messages and her own perceptions, Boikanyo said, "Since I started using the gel I feel [my herpes outbreaks] are much better. I don't know if they are really better because I am told that [the gel] is still being tested so it doesn't have any effect. But I believe that the gel is making a difference because I have seen some changes since I have started using it. . . . The gel has really helped me." Confident that she too was using an efficacious gel, another participant commented, "I think I am using 2 percent. I think it is the one that can prevent HIV. But they are not yet sure that it can prevent it and that is why they said that I have to use condoms when I use the gel." This statement hints at the second concern of MDP301 coordinators: If women believe that the gel could prevent HIV transmission, would they cease using condoms? Indeed, many women considered PRO 2000/5 to be a superior tool to condoms in preventing HIV, as issues such as dryness, breakage, and a loss of sexual pleasure were absent when using the gel. But the fears of trial coordinators proved unfounded. This was because many women viewed the primary purpose of the gel to be cleansing. HIV prevention was simply a fortunate side effect of this process. Affirming the efficacy of the gel did not result in the disuse of condoms. Trial administrators and trial participants were once again perceiving the significance of PRO 2000/5 differently.

## POTENT PARTICIPANTS

PRO 2000/5 was regarded as much more than a medication to treat vaginal infections and prevent sexually transmitted diseases. Equating cleanliness with dryness, several participants and their partners linked the gel's ability to flush contaminants and cure infections with a reduction in vaginal wetness: "I like the gel because it keeps me dry and cleanses me. I feel dry. Before I started to use the gel I used to feel like the sperms were coming out all day and my pants would be wet as a result. But when I started using the gel, it comes out with all the dirt and I remain nice and dry. The proof is I can put on panties and they stay dry." Mothudi noted, "I realized that since she started to use the gel her vagina is dry after she has washed. She is no longer as wet as she used to be. She used to have discharge that smelled bad. She used to go to the clinic for that but it never went away until she started to use the gel." As participants claimed that the gel's ability to flush pollution transformed it into a drying agent, PRO 2000/5's healing properties were linked to sexual fulfillment. Phumla stated, "I think it is the gel that encourages me to have sex more because now we are healthier." She continued, "This gel encourages me in different ways because I used to see my periods on different dates and it has cleaned my blood and my urine. I have seen that and it has improved sex between me and my partner because he used to have premature ejaculation." Beliefs regarding vaginal dryness are often equated with cleanliness (Leclerc-Madlala 2001b), and purity, health, dryness, and sexual desire are frequently imbricated. Reflecting on the changes his partner experienced while in the MDP301, Hendrick noted, "She tells me that the gel is protecting her from a lot of illnesses. . . . As a woman, it helps her a lot, especially when it comes to sex." The gel was incorporated into an embodied nexus through which sex, fidelity, pleasure, hygiene, and health were all made meaningful. Simultaneously an aphrodisiac, drying agent, and cleansing compound, PRO 2000/5 critically linked social and physiological worlds.

The gel was credited with remedying a variety of generalized physical complaints, such as muscle pains, headaches, and general feelings of malaise. A participant commented, "The gel moves around my body searching for all the ailments that I may have." Importantly, many of the ailments said to be treated by PRO 2000/5 were not explicitly associated with reproductive health. Zodwa noted, "I can wake up without feeling tired and do my washing without complaining of waist pain because before I used it my waist would be so stiff in the morning and I would not be able to work around my house." Similarly highlighting newfound strength, Zinzi stated, "I started using the gel and as a result of continuous use, my pores are now open. My body is no longer stiff and I don't get tired any more. . . . Since I started using the gel, I am always energetic like somebody who is using drugs. It has even opened the veins to my kidneys." In treating specific areas of the physical body, PRO 2000/5 improved overall well-being. After Mothudi recounted that the gel had increased his partner's vaginal dryness while curing abnormal discharge, he added, "She also started gaining weight and her face is brighter. I think the gel was doing well for her and she is happy about it." Goitsemedime noted that she too was able to gain weight and become healthier because of the cleansing properties of PRO 2000/5. Transcending specific conditions to treat the integrated person, the gel energized women and improved their lives and sense of self. Participants spoke of the gel as making them feel "complete" and "whole." One woman said, "I feel like I am a person." The ability of PRO 2000/5 to precipitate such a broad range of positive results led one participant to simply remark that it was "great for many things."

Women who praised the gel's abilities to improve their lives through cleansing and curing used it regularly and received encouragement from their partners. Hendrick recalled, "I always tell her to continue using the gel because since she has been using it, she no longer has problems with getting a heavy discharge and the gel treats her very well." The positive effects of PRO 2000/5 were said to convince even those women who had been discarding the gel to begin using it. A participant reported, "At the beginning of the study, yes, it [gel dumping] was happening, but now people no longer talk about that. Many people are saying the gel cleanses them and if a person wants to fall pregnant they use the gel for those reasons so I believe that it is no longer being dumped." Although women outside the MDP301 continued to assert that gel dumping was occurring, as the trial progressed participants contested these statements. Enrollees commented that the benefits granted by the gel—health, energy, and better sex—quickly persuaded women to overcome any doubts or hesitation that they might have initially possessed:

> Others were dumping the gel but when they heard that it was helping with this and that they started using it. They were confessing that they had been dumping the gel because they did not know what it was doing. They were saying, "Imagine inserting something I don't even know in my vagina." Others would ask us whether we are seriously using the gel and we would say yes we are using it. Then they will try it for themselves and when they come back again they will tell you that now they are using the gels and they regret dumping it in the first place.

As discussed in the previous chapter, conversations in the clinic waiting room played an important role in structuring gel use. Through these interactions, women were able to share their experiences as well as to obtain advice and guidance on a variety of matters.

One of the issues debated in the waiting room was the use of the gel outside of sexual encounters. While the trial staff instructed women to insert the gel only up to an hour before intercourse, participants wondered if it could or should be utilized at other times. For some women, the answer was yes. The belief that PRO 2000/5 flushed contaminants from female bodies led a few participants to insert it for cleaning and curing purposes regardless of their sexual activity. Some employed the gel as a medication to treat specific health problems on an as-needed basis. A participant commented, "If I feel pain in my womb I insert the gel and when it comes out it comes with dirty discharge and the pain gone." These women shared their experiences and habits. One participant described the advice she gave to a friend who was complaining of abdominal pain: "I told her to insert the gel even though she was not having sex and the following day when we spoke she said the pain has stopped and she was able to walk. She said it has removed dirt from her womb." Encouraged by these conversations and the experiences of others, a number of participants used the gel regardless of their sexual activity. While some women sought to address health concerns only when they occurred, others inserted the gel as part of their routine cleansing practices. Nomsa said, "They [trial staff] said I must insert the gel before sex but I thought it is better if I insert it even if I do not have sex because there are dirty things that come out. I use it twice a week so that it can clean me." Noting that she similarly inserted the gel even when her partner was absent, another participant asserted, "I want the gel to clean me; I want to be even cleaner. I believe that it cleans. I am sure it cleans." The general increase in energy that women experienced while on the trial also prompted regular gel use. After noting that the gel had opened her pores and the veins in her kidneys, Zinzi added, "That is what has motivated me to use the gel all the time because I am very energetic now." Perhaps the best illustration of how frequently some women used the gel occurred when a participant told us in an interview, "Even now as I am talking to you, I have it inside me."

Employing shared experiences and local conceptions of vaginal health, women independently evaluated PRO 2000/5. Despite information provided by the trial staff, women had their own criteria. While research has shown that individuals informally test the pharmaceuticals that they are prescribed, often reaching conclusions that vary from those of medical professionals (Whyte et al. 2006), PRO 2000/5 differs from over-the-counter and prescription medication in two crucial respects. First, access to the gel was tightly controlled and regimented. Potential participants had to meet a number of criteria as well as undergoing medical tests and interviews. Throughout the informed consent process, women were repeatedly told that not only was the trial placebo controlled, the efficacy of the gel was far from proven. After enrollment, women obtained new gels only after returning to the clinic each month, where these messages were reiterated. Yet within this framework, women were able to conceptualize and employ the gel in unique ways that reflected local sensibilities and habits. Furthermore, women did so through a medicalized discourse: The gel worked because it was developed through a scientific process that employed powerful chemicals tested in laboratories. Linking medical knowledge with popular narratives, Zodwa said:

> I think [PRO 2000/5] has been thoroughly researched and herbs of high quality have been used to produce this gel so that it can help women. The people who have produced this really know a woman's body and what it needs, because there are many diseases and women are mostly vulnerable to them and they knew that the gel will work on the areas in a woman's body that have been damaged by those diseases, especially sexual feelings, and this brings a major change to women who have not been enjoying sex.

In asserting the efficacy of PRO 2000/5, women made their own meaning despite repeated messages to the contrary. While pharmaceutical companies, governments, and research organizations control a great deal of the development and parameters of a trial, MDP301 participants were not passive subjects. Rather than submitting uncritically to trial apparatus and messages, women created their own medical narratives, which situated PRO 2000/5 within existing sensibilities of pollution, sexuality, and health.

As participants discussed the ability of the gel to increase fertility, treat infections, or prevent HIV, trial staff had no way to contest these declarations. Unlike licensed pharmaceuticals, PRO 2000/5 had yet to be proven effective. While clinic staff did not agree with participants' claims of efficacy, they could not easily dismiss them. A clinical trial is one instance in which biomedical knowledge is notably uncertain. As a double-blind trial, the MDP301 could not refute women's claims over which of the three gels they had been assigned. Likewise, doctors reported that the gel should not have an effect on conception, but as it had yet to be extensively tested, they could not decisively make this assurance. In the absence of substantive medical evidence, women's voices could not be comprehensively challenged. Consequently, through the process of participating in MDP301, women gained legitimacy for their experiences and beliefs not only within the community but also in the trial. With limited data on hand regarding in vivo use, medical professionals and trial staff relied on the participants to gather information about the gel. Throughout the MDP301, women were regularly interviewed and their opinions about the gel were repeatedly sought. Told that the success of the trial rested on their gel use, participants came to realize that their experiences granted them a knowledge that researchers did not possess. This awareness reshaped the relationship between researchers and researched. Conscious of their role as evaluators, trial participants commented that doctors were now dependent on undereducated and economically disadvantaged black women. Basing their claims on this unique knowledge, MDP301 participants stated that they knew what trial researchers did not—the gel worked.

# The Biotechnical Salvation of a Failed Pharmaceutical

6

As the MDP301 progressed, more and more participants asserted that the gel worked. Even as trial staff reminded participants that PRO 2000/5 had yet to be proven effective, they too felt confident in a positive result. A smaller, earlier trial of PRO 2000/5 had shown efficacy, and many staff on the MDP301 felt that it would be the first truly successful microbicide trial in history. However, even before the end of the trial, troubling signs appeared. In February 2008, the Independent Data Monitoring Committee (IDMC) for the MDP301 recommended that the evaluation of 2 percent PRO 2000/5 gel be discontinued, as there was "no more than a small chance of it showing protection against HIV infection" (Gafos et al. 2011). As women on the 2 percent arm were informed and asked to turn in their gels, trialists and participants continued to have faith in PRO 2000/5. In an effort to spread the message of microbicides to a wider audience, the MDP301 conducted a workshop where participants collaborated with musicians to produce a song about the trial. In the final cut, listeners were urged to "hold on" to the promise of microbicides. However, a few months later, the hopes of trialists and participants were dashed. After reviewing the data from all five sites, the MDP301 reported that PRO 2000/5 gel was safe to use but ineffective in preventing HIV transmission (McCormack et al. 2010).

For many, the trial seemed to be a failure, but the MDP301 was adamant that this was not the case. From a scientific perspective, trials that are able to produce a result are successful, whether the results are negative or positive. Microbicide scientists and trialists thus prefer not to use the word "failure" to describe unsuccessful trials. But a reluctance to admit failure does not merely reflect a concern for scientific accuracy: "Widely considered to be the pathway to objectivity in modern biomedical research, clinical trial results in practice may be subject to considerable amounts of interpretative flexibility. Precisely because the stakes are often high—both in human lives and in stock market values—the deciphering of clinical trial findings may prove not only a contentious process, but also a highly public one" (Epstein 1997:691). Rather than focusing on PRO 2000/5's lack of efficacy, the MDP301 press releases and public statements concentrated on the positive outcomes—such as HIV testing for women and capacity building—and argued that the trial had conclusively proved that microbicides have the power to improve women's lives. Although they had found PRO 2000/5 to be an ineffective product, advocates and trialists sought to keep the dream of microbicides alive.

For participants, the trial results came as a severe blow. Throughout the course of the MDP301, its protocols—regular HIV testing, health checks, and counseling—had improved women's confidence. "Strength" and "control" were two common words in participants' descriptions of what they had gained on the trial. These narratives increasingly used religious themes and iconography. Participants spoke of sacrificing their health for the trial, having faith in the gel, and experiencing salvation as a result. Clinical trial participation was said to have saved them. However, their strength and control disappeared with the end of the MDP301 and the release of the results. Deprived of clinical visits, HIV testing, and faith in PRO 2000/5, the women's lives returned to what they had been prior to their involvement in the trial. In praising microbicides as an empowering technology, advocates and trialists failed to realize that it was the trial itself that had precipitated change.

## LOSING AN ARM

In February 2008, the MDP301's IDMC met to review the progress of the trial and to assess any safety concerns. IDMCs make decisions and recommendations regarding the continuity of clinical trials and may halt a trial or part of a trial if they see that the drug being evaluated is significantly effective, if there are safety issues, or if it is apparent that efficacy will not be demonstrated (Gafos et al. 2011). Based on the data collected, the IDMC for the MDP301 trial recommended halting the 2 percent arm immediately. With little or no difference in HIV infections between the placebo and the 2 percent product arm, the IDMC concluded that it would be futile to continue this component of the trial. The MDP301 steering committee agreed that trial participants randomized to the 2 percent arm should be exited from the trial. Although there was an option to reallocate them to the 0.5 percent arm, the trial coordinators felt that this might undermine the validity of the randomization schedule (ibid.). Plans were drawn up to inform the affected participants at study visits, during community activities, and over the phone.[1] At the Johannesburg site, a total of 767 women had been randomized to the 2 percent gel. However, 393 of these women had either completed their enrollment or withdrawn for various reasons, leaving 374 participants to track. Once informed, women were instructed to return their unused gels; although they would no longer be using the product, these participants would have their health monitored for three months as part of a safety assessment.

While trial administrators justified the cessation of the 2 percent arm in terms of statistical benchmarks, a lack of proven efficacy, and biomedical expediency, community members and trial participants expressed a variety of responses that drew from and capitalized on prevailing narratives regarding PRO 2000. For many, the cancellation of the 2 percent arm raised two key questions: Why was a stronger concentration of the drug less effective than a weaker version? Was there any evidence that the higher dose of PRO 2000/5 might have caused harm to participants? Conscious that the early closure of other microbicide trials was often due to a potentially injurious product, the MDP301 initiated an education campaign to disseminate information and to reassure continuing participants that PRO 2000/5 was not a health risk. Despite the trial's desire to dispel community concerns definitively, its answers were at times ambiguous. The official "Q and A" document published on the MDP website states:

### 9. How can a stronger dose of product be less effective than a weaker dose?

We don't know the answer to that but are planning to investigate further. It is biologically plausible that a product may show no protective effect against HIV infection at a concentration of 2%, but show a protective effect at a lower concentration (0.5%). There are a number of possible explanations for this, one being that any beneficial effect against HIV could be partly outweighed by a local effect on the vaginal lining related to the higher concentration product. In other words, the weaker dose may be gentler on the vagina.

**10. Does that mean that the stronger dose (2%) may have caused harm to the women who received it?**

The reason given by the DMC for their recommendation to discontinue the 2% PRO 2000/5 arm was that there was no more than a small chance of it showing protection. This indicates that there was no conclusive evidence of harm or increased risk of infection in those women who had received 2% PRO 2000/5. (MDP 2008:1)

These responses seemed to ask questions rather than give answers. Perhaps most notably, the IDMC seemed only to imply that PRO 2000/5 was safe rather than making an explicit statement to this effect. While community members and participants expected clear and concise answers, this was something that the MDP301 was to some extent incapable of producing at this stage. Cessation of the 2 percent arm was based on statistics, and until further investigations occurred, more definitive answers were simply not available.

Given the lack of concrete information, MDP301 staff attempted to inform the public strategically of the closure. In the past, the trial had used Theta FM and similar stations to promote participation, and this platform was now utilized to disseminate information about the fate of the 2 percent arm. To supplement these broadcasts, a series of public meetings was also conducted. However, even weeks after radio announcements and community meetings, many were unaware of what had occurred. For those who did hear of the changes to the trial, the information was often unclear. Initially, clinic workers and community advisory board members were unable to articulate responses to many of the questions they received at these meetings and required the presence of clinical staff to assist them. As anticipated, Sowetans and Orange Farmers were anxious that PRO 2000/5 had been found to be toxic. At a community advisory board meeting, members asked if the gel was in fact a "poison" that would encourage HIV transmission. These anxieties drew from pervasive narratives stressing the malevolence of the trial; the closure of the 2 percent arm seemed to give credence to the rumors. Despite repeated denials from staff, a number of people said that the discontinuation clearly demonstrated not only that the gel contained HIV but that the MDP301 was nothing more than a plot to kill Africans. Some residents proclaimed that they at last had proof for what they had always suspected. As a result, family, friends, and neighbors of trial participants on the other arms urged them to withdraw immediately. To discourage rumors, some participants chose not to tell those outside the trial. While a few outspoken community members accused the trial of wrongdoing, their stance did not achieve widespread popularity. Unlike the CS trial, the media did not report the closing of the 2 percent arm, and the MDP301 was not publicly accused of harming African women.

Nevertheless, these rumors, coupled with the cessation of the 2 percent arm, were extremely disturbing for some women. According to a number of participants, the IDMC had actually determined that the 2 percent gel made women vulnerable to HIV infection, despite the assurances of the MDP301. Believing that there was a higher incidence of seroconversion among women on the 2 percent arm, a few participants compared the MDP301 to the CS trials in KwaZulu-Natal. However, many others stated that this comparison was simply false, noting their persistent status as HIV negative. When Zinzi saw women on the 2 percent arm returning their gels at the clinic, she did not worry about her ongoing enrollment. Once she returned home, Zinzi informed her partner of the closure, explaining that while the arm had been halted because the gel was ineffective, they were not in danger of becoming infected with HIV or suffering other adverse effects. After asking her a few questions, he accepted her explanation and agreed that she should continue participating in the MDP301.

Although HIV risk was regularly dismissed, participants, worried about other complications the gel could cause. Having received her initial notification by phone, one participant feared getting another call in a few weeks or months informing her that irreparable damage to her body had occurred. Another described turning in her gels at the clinic and feeling confident when she left, only to begin having doubts once she returned home. She became so fretful that she consulted a private doctor, who conducted an examination. Although the doctor detected nothing amiss, she was still scared that a "long-term side effect" could result from her gel use. For others, the discontinuation reinforced beliefs that the trial was fundamentally concerned about participants' health. One participant noted that the closure proved the trial was responsibly employing specialists who were consistently reviewing the data being collected and immediately recommending protocol changes when any issues were identified. She added that she now had even more faith in the trial than previously. During a focus group, several participants remarked that they "felt great" about the trial taking action and notifying them in a timely manner. It showed that participants were "always protected."

When refuting rumors of harm, participants regularly blamed other enrollees. In one instance, we were told, "People are saying that . . . it [the closure] means 2 percent gel has infected many women with HIV, but I told them that when we join the study we were told that we should use the gel with a condom because they don't know if the gel prevents HIV or not so if some women didn't use the gel with a condom, it is their fault, not researchers.'" Rather than focusing on PRO 2000/5 or trial protocols, this participant blamed others for using the gel in an unsafe manner. Statements such as hers were common, hardening accusations against women in the trial who were suspected of nonuse or improper use of the gel. An anonymous comment posted in the suggestion box at the clinic read: "It is unfair for people like us who had just started to use the [2 percent] gel because of people who were not willing to use it properly. Please do something for us." Some women were thought not to use the gel because they were afraid of inserting an untested substance into their vaginas, but many others were accused of joining the trial solely for personal gain. Participants on the 2 percent arm often brought up the problem of "greedy women" who were motivated by cash. One added, "Most women are not using the gel and they are telling each other to participate in these studies so they can get R150."

Throughout focus groups and interviews examining participants' responses to the discontinuation, women characterized gel dumpers as "naughty" and blamed them for endangering the scientific process. Wanting to remain on the trial, several women asked to be given the gels of dumpers: "Some of them dump the gel because they only need the money that they get from the study. And I have even asked them to give me the gels instead of dumping them because I needed them and I was disappointed after they stopped me from using the gels." Dumping was seen to be "wrong" because it threatened the trial and hindered the "fight" against HIV. Some women even urged the trial to inspect women's bodies to ensure that they were using the gel. Without these checks, the trial was a "waste of time" because so much gel had been discarded unused that not even the 0.5 percent arm would prove effective. After the closure, many feared that the entire trial could end early and placed the blame squarely on irresponsible gel dumpers. Mosa said, "If the study fails because of this gel dumping then the study will close. What about those people who are using the gel? It means they are going to be affected because of those who did not use the gel." Gel dumping also provided a coherent explanation for why a stronger concentration of PRO 2000/5 had been found ineffective. It was reasoned that this arm had had a high percentage of gel dumpers, and that their skewing of the data was the primary reason for the arm's early closure. Yet for others the very fact that a result had been announced proved that the gel was being utilized. One participant said, "This finding shows that the study is making progress and it shows that participants were using the gel in order for there to be a finding." This led to speculation that the 0.5 percent gel would be found to be effective.

Whether caused by gel dumpers or an ineffective product, the lack of efficacy in the 2 percent gel generated widespread feelings of disappointment. Several participants said they had "lost hope" in the MDP301. When Glory was first told the news, she "panicked," worried that the 0.5 percent gel also wasn't working. When she told her partner, "He didn't say anything; he only responded with a sigh." For women on the 2 percent arm, there was a sense that their participation had been a waste of time, while those on the remaining arms wondered if there was any point to their gel use, particularly given the possibility that the entire trial could close early. While some felt that the 0.5 percent gel would also prove a failure, others refused to give up. Many women said that it was important that the trial persist "so that a cure can be found eventually," reflecting ongoing hope in the efficacy of the 0.5 percent gel. To help in this effort, women on the 2 percent arm often expressed a desire to be reallocated to one of the other arms. While they were motivated by a desire to assist in finding an effective product, they also sought continued access to the gel.

Given the presumed positive effects of PRO 2000/5, women on the 2 percent arm were anxious that their health would diminish without it. A community health worker responsible for exiting participants randomized to the 2 percent arm noted this trend, adding that the gel "had done something good in their bodies." Throughout their exit interviews, participants repeatedly commented on the gel's positive effects, noting that it was much more than just a potential HIV prevention tool. A number of women reported using the gel outside of sexual intercourse to cleanse their vaginas or to treat health complaints such as abdominal pain. One woman asserted that despite repeatedly applying metronidazole to treat a heavy and foul-smelling vaginal discharge, she had not seen a sustained improvement until she began using the gel. The gel had also allowed her to enjoy sex with her partner in a way she had not experienced previously. Given these effects, she had no concerns about the safety of the product. Describing her reaction to the closure of the 2 percent arm, she said, "I am angry and I am sad." She was not alone. In one focus group discussion, all the participants present reported that the gel had enhanced their pleasure during sex while cleansing their bodies and protecting them from infection. They described how PRO 2000/5 killed STIs while being "friendly" to a man's sperm, thus encouraging conception. After learning that the 2 percent concentration was ineffective in preventing HIV infection, they did not reevaluate these beliefs. In fact, participants noted that they would persist in using the gel simply for its cleansing and aphrodisiac properties. In a telling sign, two of the women present had yet to return their unused gels to the clinic. For many women, improvements in sex and health had resulted in happier and more secure lives. Consequently, women worried that their quality of life would diminish without access to the gel.

Rather than fundamentally shifting views about the trial or PRO 2000/5, the cessation of the 2 percent arm often reinforced existing opinions. Although the MDP301 tried to guide discourse about the closure through the dissemination of information, this had little effect. Narratives of traditional men and greedy women pervaded participant and community discussions. Those who had seen the MDP301 as a tool of malicious genocidal whites felt the closure had proved their assertions, while others dismissed these accusations as ignorance. And even though the trial had shown that the 2 percent gel did not prevent HIV infection, women remained insistent that the gel was effective as a cleansing agent and aphrodisiac. Trial staff responded to these narratives as they had before, claiming that the views of participants and community members indicated a "knowledge gap." When unenrolled participants asked why they were not moved to the 0.5 percent arm, it indicated to the principal investigator their "poor comprehension" of the randomization procedures. We observed her telling the community health workers to continue educating participants about the scientific rationale for randomization as follows: "If they fail to remember the key messages, we repeat educating them about the key messages and encourage them to revise [review] the study information sheet so that they know about the study's key messages. We also document the information in the source documents." Rather than reevaluating their communication methods, MDP301 staff simply portrayed participants as ignorant and reiterated the same standardized information. Through its key messages, the trial sought to control meaning but was repeatedly unable to do so.

## A TRIAL WITHOUT A PHARMACEUTICAL

The closure fundamentally altered trial participation for women using the 2 percent gel. Rather than being removed from the trial completely, they were informed that they would be monitored for another three months. For many, this somewhat relieved the disappointment of exiting the arm. As women began turning in their gels, they often remarked that they were pleased that they would "continue to be taken care of" by the trial. While participants were no longer using the gel, they still had monthly appointments, underwent HIV tests and health screenings, and were interviewed by trial staff. Although social scientists and medical researchers tend to cast the purpose of trials strictly in terms pharmaceutical testing, this is only one aspect of much larger projects. Disentangling the MDP301 from PRO 2000/5 reveals that many women not only conceptualized the trial as distinct from the gel but also tended to value the former just as much if not more than the latter. One woman said that it was important for her to participate in the MDP301 "not only because of the gel, but also because I am always up to date with my health status." Another participant said, "Before I came to join the study I didn't understand HIV/AIDS, but now I understand it. As women there are things that we are insensitive about because there are things we don't care much about. But coming to this clinic I learned to take care of myself because the study is not only about the gel but we also get help." For many, this help included assistance with monitoring reproductive health, ascertaining HIV status, and successfully encouraging condom use.

In reviewing trial outcomes, MDP301 coordinators found that through HIV testing and counseling, participants were increasingly able to convince their partners to wear condoms. Like many women, Boikanyo and Nomsa both said that they had not been condom users prior to the trial, but they had changed their behavior after speaking to nurses. This trend was echoed throughout the trial. Furthermore, linking the primary task of participants—gel use—with condoms prompted women to regard condom use as mandatory: "When you use the gel you must use the condom. So that thing forced me to use condoms most of the time but there were fewer times when I did not use a condom." Similarly, Zinzi noted that because the gel and condoms "work together," she began using condoms for the first time, having previously avoided them for fear of infectious worms. A number of women on the 2 percent arm announced that they would like to participate in future studies because the trial had taught them to successfully insist on condoms. One commented, "I learned to be responsible because before I joined the study I didn't care much about condoms but since I joined the study I have learned to use them." For some like Boikanyo, the counseling provided by the trial led them to be more assertive, openly discussing sexual issues with their partners. For others, filling out the coital diary drew attention to when and how they had sex as well as their condom habits: "It [the diary] also helps me because before I joined the study, I was never aware or conscious about how many times I had sex. The diary has also given me the confidence to use condoms consistently." Precious similarly noted that having to record when she did and did not use a condom motivated her to employ prophylaxis regularly.

While MDP301 coordinators and participants tended to focus on direct linkages between trial procedures and a decrease in risk behavior, in some cases women tactically exploited popular rumors regarding the gel. Concerned that the gel was potentially toxic, some men began using condoms without being prompted. Hendrick, for instance, had been resistant, complaining that condoms caused discomfort and bloating. But this changed during the trial. His partner, Andiswa, noted that he is now the one suggesting that they use condoms. In a few cases, participants warned their partners that the gel could cause men pain or injury. After hinting that the gel produced a penile rash, Nobuhle no longer had difficulty convincing her partner to wear a condom. Wanting this behavior to endure past the end of the trial, Nobuhle informed him that she would be using the gel for three years, not one. Nobuhle misled her partner to create the outcome she desired. Although few women lied to their partners like Nobuhle, they similarly relied on the trial to ensure condom usage. Our data shows that once women left the MDP301, they were less likely to insist on condom use and their partners tended to have more resistance to the practice. Rather than a behavior that couples continued, increased condom utilization was confined to the trial.

Perhaps the most important aspect of the MDP301 was HIV testing. After their initial enrollment, participants were screened for HIV every three months; they praised the trial for these tests. The comments of participants were so positive that a member of the clinic staff suggested that the MDP301 clinics could function as an alternative voluntary HIV counseling and testing center. This was in part because HIV tests were difficult if not impossible to get elsewhere. While a few participants vowed to attend public health clinics once their enrollment ended, most were skeptical of this option. Nomsa said that she would never get tested at a public clinic because the nurses there were "horrible." Another participant was more specific, saying, "You are not free to get tested because you see people who have just tested for HIV and the next day you would hear people saying so and so is HIV positive. How did they know? It is obvious that they were told by people who tested you." Like this participant, many did not trust the public health sector to keep results confidential. Others complained that these clinics were overcrowded and unhygienic and employed rude staff. In contrast, the MDP301 clinics were thought to be clean and reliable: "What I like most about this [MDP301] clinic is that whenever I have a blood test done I know that there are no chances of me having direct contact with somebody else's blood because hygiene is a priority, unlike at a public clinic. I am certain that if the blood test results came back saying I was HIV positive, then that would mean that I really am HIV positive." Indeed, South Africa's public health care system is severely strained and client care is notoriously weak, particularly in townships such as Soweto and Orange Farm. As a result, community clinics were reluctant to expend treatment resources unnecessarily. Although HIV testing was promoted throughout South Africa, in reality these tests were often given only to women perceived to be "high risk." Women over the age of 35 noted that some community clinic nurses refused to test them for HIV, saying that they were too old to have sex and therefore not at risk. Others were tested only once, and were told by nursing staff that further tests were unnecessary when they returned a few months later. In contrast to public health clinics, the trial clinics were praised as supportive and ideal testing locations.

Trial coordinators acknowledged the importance of providing regular testing, hoping it would prevent the unintended infection of others and ensure that HIV-positive individuals received treatment promptly. Couched in these terms, testing was thought to reduce "risky" behavior, and this was certainly the case. However, portraying testing as simply a tool to encourage condom use or early treatment for HIV often overlooks the profound fear and social stigma attached to HIV in South Africa (Mills 2006; Petros et al. 2006; Robins 2006). While epidemiologists discussed prevalence rates, South

Africans were struggling to come to terms with a disease decimating families across the country. Participants repeatedly described their sorrow, anger, and confusion as friends and family members fell ill and died. Upset by the death of her sister, who had refused to admit that she had AIDS, and reflecting on her own vulnerability, Sesi said:

> I worried that if I should get sick, I would get sicker than my sister because she was ill for three years. And I thought, it means that I will probably be sicker than my sister, so I must know now while there's still time. . . . She leaves two children, and I thought, I also have two children, so if I stay without knowing where I stand, what's going to happen to my children when I die? . . . Even today, her children have no idea what was wrong with their mother. And it is so painful.

Stories such as Sesi's were told by many women across South Africa. Like her sister, many choose to keep their diagnosis secret, while others refused testing altogether. The stigma, fear, and suffering associated with HIV formed a powerful backdrop to the MDP301. Sesi said, "That is why I was happy to come here because here I can test for AIDS and all these other diseases because these days we don't know what kills and what doesn't kill. These diseases all kill." Given the fear and uncertainty of the HIV threat, the MDP301 was much more than a reliable method to discover one's status. Testing was a frightening but life-altering experience.

Uniformly nervous when faced with their initial HIV test, participants gained confidence after repeated testing. Like Mandisa, women felt relief after the first test showed that they were HIV negative, but they remained apprehensive. Worried that they were merely in the window period, when HIV antibodies are still undetectable, participants experienced anxiety as their second test approached. However, as their HIV negative status endured, these fears began to dissipate. Khentsani recalled, "I thought maybe the virus was still hiding in my body. So when I got tested the second time I was reassured that I do not have it. My responsibility was to be careful and focus on one partner." Like many participants, Khentsani noted that each time she was tested, her confidence increased. Boikanyo commented, "I don't get scared anymore when I have to take some blood tests. I don't even imagine that I might find out that I am HIV positive." For the overwhelming majority of participants, this was not a false confidence. At the end of the trial, 95.6

percent (2,393 of 2,503 women) of the Johannesburg participants had remained HIV negative throughout their enrollment.[2] For these women, repeated testing continually confirmed their status. As enrollment was contingent upon remaining HIV negative, the two became conflated. Being an MDP301 participant meant staying free of HIV and healthy. As a result, being a trial participant became a powerful identity; the trial created a space where women exercised knowledge and control of their bodies.

Participants repeatedly affirmed that their status led them to take their health much more seriously. Having demonstratively avoided HIV thus far, women began working earnestly to maintain their status. Reflecting on her time in the trial, Boikanyo recalled:

> Before I started participating in the study, I was just sitting at home and I was not doing any blood tests or medical exams. I didn't know exactly what was happening with me. That sometimes can make you reckless with your life because you keep telling yourself that it doesn't matter how you behave as you might already be infected anyway. But the minute you discover that you are HIV negative, then you feel lucky to be still HIV negative and you don't want to ever spoil that for yourself.

Linking testing, the MDP301, and a strong desire to avoid HIV, women praised the trial for positively changing their attitudes. Boikanyo continued, "The study is about making a difference in your life and it reminds you that you need to take better care of yourself as a person. I think the study has saved a lot of people who would have otherwise become infected had they not joined the study and followed the study requirements." The MDP301's tests motivated participants to "take care" of themselves. Boikanyo said that after she tested HIV negative at her initial screening, "I told myself that I was going to stay like that by being faithful to one partner. The study gave me the confidence to take control of my life and helped me make the decision to live. My life has been good ever since I started participating in the study." Transcending HIV, the trial not only improved women's health through testing; it encouraged women to monitor and maintain their healthy bodies proactively. In these narratives, female agency was made real through trial participation. As women repeatedly tested negative, medical procedures confirmed that their efforts to take care of themselves were successful. Participants worried that without such proof, they would abandon regular testing, condom use, and other steps to ensure that they remained HIV negative. Consequently, women on the 2 percent arm expressed relief when being informed that they would continue to be observed by the trial. After talking to one such participant, a member of the clinic staff said, "She sees not being dropped from the study as a motivating factor to continue 'looking after herself' like she was when she was still using the gel and following study procedures." While women enjoyed gel use, cessation of the 2 percent arm revealed that the most critical aspects of the trial for many participants were health monitoring and HIV testing.

Given the stigma of HIV, being able to claim an HIV negative identity consistently became an expression of morality. Throughout South Africa, women and men feared contracting HIV from unfaithful partners, particularly as condoms were eschewed in long-term monogamous relationships. Linking disease with promiscuity, women transformed HIV testing into a method of monitoring fidelity. Discussing her initial attitude toward receiving an HIV test, a participant remarked, "I was not afraid because I have not been doing bad things." Acknowledging the moral connotations of HIV, a number of churches in and around Johannesburg conducted testing as a part of spiritual assessment and outreach. Parishioners revealed to be HIV negative were congratulated and told not to change their virtuous ways. Trial participants capitalized on these notions, noting that their continued status as HIV negative proved their faithfulness, asserting their morality to their partners. Stating that the MDP301 had greatly helped her, Sihle described the self-assurance she derived from repeatedly reporting her health to her partner. She said, "It means he knows that I am a woman who likes HIV testing. It means the study has made me strong, not to be afraid to check my HIV status, and I even tell him that I am going to check my HIV status." In noting that she likes testing and informs her partner in advance, Sihle displays confidence in her behavior and well-being.

Invoking their identity as HIV negative, participants differentiated themselves from other women in Soweto and Orange Farm. Whereas women in the trial referred to themselves as "healthy," those outside the trial were labeled "cowards" and "lazy." A participant said, "We are different because if you join the study it means you are responsible about your life. So those who did not join the study, they do not care about their life." These statements often revolved around the presumed unwillingness of nonparticipants to be screened for HIV. Fear of HIV testing was invoked as proof that nonparticipants were promiscuous and, as a result, could not be trusted. It was these immoral individuals who were said to be responsible for spreading inaccurate rumors about the trial. After participating in the trial for only a month, Kagiso commented, "Women who are promiscuous say bad things about the clinic. . . . Some say that the gel will infect women with HIV because they are paying women who are using the gel. And I do not believe what they are saying because they know that they have multiple partners and that is why they say all these things." Similarly, another trial participant speculated that the blood-selling rumor was spread by HIV-positive women who had been excluded from the trial: "They are lying. These are people who are HIV positive and cannot get into the study. They are just jealous." Through these statements, participants not only refuted narratives labeling them as greedy, immoral women using the trial for financial gain; they inverted them. These counternarratives acted as a powerful rejoinder to public accusations of impropriety. A participant said that when she community members told her that she would die "for the sake of getting R150, I tell them that I am better because I know my health and I am even aware of my HIV status."

Rejecting accusations of greed, participants reframed trial enrollment as evidence of altruism. Referring to themselves as "volunteers" and "lifesavers," participants stressed that their involvement in the trial was moral because it benefited society at large. Volunteers stated that their participation was for the collective good rather than individual profit, and that it assisted others beyond their testing of a potentially lifesaving pharmaceutical. A primary focus of these narratives was blood selling. As discussed in the third chapter, some Sowetans and Orange Farmers believed that routine blood draws were in fact a way for the MDP301 to extract and sell the blood of participants, thereby exploiting poor African women. Simultaneously building on and transforming these rumors, participants acknowledged that they did receive money for their blood, but insisted that it was because they were HIV negative. They concluded that the clinics were donating their "good," uninfected blood to health facilities and private individuals who required it for transfusions: "They are saying we are being paid this R150 because we are donating our blood which you then take to Baragwanath Hospital to give other people who need it." In this story, participants' blood was given to others but the reimbursements were not payment in the strict sense, but part of a reciprocal exchange. Furthermore, participant blood was "helping people" who needed blood transfusions or were ill. Although she did not enjoy having her blood drawn so frequently and in such large quantities, one participant nevertheless commented, "I like one thing [about giving blood]: Maybe my blood is going to work for someone who is sick, you see." Another participant succinctly said, "It is good for my blood to save someone's life." Not only did their HIV-negative identity mark participants as virtuous, this status reportedly benefited others through their donated blood. Women invoked trial procedures such as HIV testing and blood draws as powerful assertions of their own virtue and integrity.

Reinforcing these stories of their selflessness, participants transformed cash reimbursements for blood from a dangerous and selfish act into part of a long-term productive relationship between the clinical trial and its enrollees. We were told that the reimbursements were intended to serve as part of exchanges that benefited those in need, rather than payments in the strict sense of the term. In this narrative, cash for blood was portrayed altruistically. Furthermore, the money received by the women supported the wider social unit. Nomsa, for instance, stressed that she used her reimbursement to purchase clothes for her child. Trial participants emphasized that they spent cash from the trial not on fashionable clothes or perfumes, but on vegetables and meat (including liver), which nurtured entire families while also replenishing their own blood. Just as accusations of blood stealing resembled charges against the illicit actions of witches, rumors of blood selling echoed legitimate instances of blood exchanged for cash, such as transactions of bridewealth, where cash is given for a woman's reproductive potential, or metaphorically, for her blood. Like *lobola*, "donating" blood at the trial clinic was framed as an instance in which the exchange of cash for blood engendered legitimate bonds. The participants' insistence that they were involved in a reciprocal relationship with the clinic—a cyclical flow of lifesaving blood for blood-renewing cash—transformed what some viewed as an amoral act of consumption into a model of social and procreative relations. The women's acceptance of money for blood was not an attack on the very basis of relatedness; instead, the women claimed to be cultivating life, health, and personhood through their participation in the MDP301.

Interestingly, HIV testing and the frequency with which it was conducted were ostensibly designed to provide the data needed to assess the efficacy of PRO 2000/5. Testing was not optional, but rather a required component of trial participation. As one participant said, "The ticket for entering the study is you have to test the blood." Given that HIV tests were mandatory for all trial participants, it is certainly possible to consider them a form of bio-control, in which women were prohibited from refusing or resisting the tests. From this perspective, the MDP301 regulated women's bodies for the benefit of the pharmaceutical industry. Clinical trials have routinely been cast as oppressive, but in so doing, the multivocality of medical procedures is ignored. Rather than viewing the steady screenings as procedures imposed on women's bodies, participants praised them. Noting that fear and inconvenience would have dissuaded them from repeated testing, they admitted initially submitting to the tests only because it was a requirement for enrollment. But apprehension gave way to confidence as their HIV status was confirmed month after month. Consequently, the trial procedures themselves became a source of power for trial participants. Women invoked HIV testing and status to alter their social positionality dramatically. On one hand, women felt in control of their bodies and, as a result, their selves. On the other, adopting an HIV-negative identity allowed women to assert their virtue to sexual partners and community members.

## "HOLD ON"

Participants' opinions of the MDP301 and PRO 2000/5 were given voice during a weeklong workshop designed by coordinators in an attempt to disseminate trial messages to a wider audience. During the workshop, which was held between the discontinuation of the 2 percent arm in February 2008 and the official announcement of the final trial results in December 2009, former MDP301 participants and emerging musicians from Orange Farm and Soweto composed a pop song about the MDP301. The production was funded by a Wellcome Trust International Engagement Award, a grant to communicate and popularize scientific research by promoting social exchanges between science and the arts. Twenty-five former trial participants were invited to narrate their experiences of the trial, while thirteen local musicians assisted them in constructing lyrical interpretations and providing musical content. With the theme of "There Is a Song in My Story," the workshop was intended to encourage participants to contribute oral and written accounts of their experiences in the trial while the musicians listened and produced multiple drafts of the song. Seeking to acknowledge the perspectives of participants, as well as to create a song that would appeal to a wide range of Sowetans and Orange Farmers, the MDP301 chose *kwaito* as the genre. *Kwaito*, a style developed in Johannesburg, resembles house and hip-hop music while using African sounds and samples. Possessing percussive and melodic loops as well as deep bass lines, *kwaito* often has a slower tempo range than other forms of house music. Distinctively sung, shouted, and rapped, *kwaito* lyrics are created out of the experiences of everyday township life. *Kwaito*, a Tsotsitaal word, is derived from the Afrikaans *kwai*, which traditionally meant "angry" but is now used colloquially to denote something that is cool or hip. Born out of urban experiences of economic marginalization and ethnic blending, *kwaito* gives township residents a mainstream voice.

After the workshop, the musicians edited a final version of the song, which was recorded and then played on local radio stations.[3] Predictably, the lyrics of the song (written mostly in isiZulu) focused a great deal on standardized trial information. Seeking to communicate the purpose of the trial and those who are eligible to enroll, one verse exhorts:

> *Eqondane ngqo na labo abazitika ngoko cantsi*
> *Kodwa abanganalo igciwane lekagawulayo*
> *Uzocwaningisiswa kahle ukuthi ingasithiba na isifo socantsi.*
> *Eish! Kodwa abancelisayo*
> *Hai kabe one side,*
> *Hai kabe one side*

> It is aimed at those who are sexually active
> But not those who are infected with HIV
> It is being researched to see if it can prevent STIs.
> Oh! But those who are breastfeeding
> Sorry you are excluded,
> Sorry you are excluded.

As this illustrates, the song was an additional vehicle to publicize the MDP301's key messages. In another verse, the song states that the gel is "a friend to the condom" and urges couples to use both technologies concurrently. For many MDP301 staff, the song was another method of providing information in a form that they assumed would be approachable and intelligible for Sowetans and Orange Farmers. Indeed, participants commented that the song parroted much of what they had been told throughout the recruitment process. However, there were some segments of the song that were much more open to interpretation.

While most of the song's lines were devoted to educating listeners about the trial, a few sought to express the views and voices of participants, most notably in an early draft of the chorus:

> *Noma ku nzima*
> *Ungalahlithemba*
> *Bambelela*
> *Qinisela*

> Even if it's hard
> Don't lose hope
> Hold on
> Hold on tight

Seeking to convey hopeful anticipation, the chorus urged listeners to be optimistic about an eventual solution to the AIDS crisis in South Africa. Although this message was articulated by many who heard the song, there was debate over exactly what one should hold on to. This ambiguity, like the uncertainness of the gel itself, encouraged listeners to draw their own conclusions. For some, the chorus was an admonition to hold onto the promise of pharmaceuticals. One woman said, "To me this chorus—*Bambelela*—is like they are saying there is still hope that there are medications that are being tested that might still prevent HIV." This perspective was echoed by another woman: "The lyrics of the song are saying 'hold on,' they will find that thing. 'Hold on' means that we don't have to lose hope; we have to keep hoping that prevention will be found." In making statements about the potential power of microbicides, others explicitly associated hope with gendered aspirations. Not only would a microbicide assist in preventing HIV, it would also allow women to take control of their bodies:

> I feel that maybe the song says that women should hold on to the hope that women also will have something that belongs to them. Without

depending on men, like if I am told that it is raining you should bring a raincoat [condom]. If this gel works then I will just shoot my gel and keep quiet. It is my responsibility, it is my life, it is my body, and I don't have to depend on someone for what it is mine.

Noting that female independence from men was a significant outcome of participation, some women criticized the song for failing to articulate this experience clearly. One participant said that the song lacked "the message that women should empower themselves, own their bodies, and be responsible. You don't have to say that my husband does not like it. It is my life. It is my body. Women need to be empowered and when there are studies they must participate and get involved. That boosts confidence." Although lyrics focusing on female empowerment were absent from the final version of the song, they were repeatedly voiced during the workshop. Shifting from the official version of the song to the many drafts composed during the workshop reveals the depth of women's experiences during the MDP301. Rather than reiterating the key trial messages, participants described their enrollment as transformative: joining the trial as fearful women, they had risked their lives to ultimately achieve salvation.

Participants' life-changing journeys through the trial were narrated from the very beginning of the workshop. Asked to identify several themes that they felt characterized their participation in the MDP301, women listed: *truth, fear, in control, sacrifice, courage, curiosity, from bad to good, opportunity, overcoming adversity, pride, hope, uncertainty, improved sex, waiting—celebrate,* and *feeling good.* They were then asked to draw from this list to compose lyrics that could potentially be used as a chorus for the song. After a general discussion, the following lines were proposed:

| Concept | Lyrics |
| --- | --- |
| Truth | It is true that we are dying |
| Courage | I got courageous to take a test |
| In control | Now I'm in control of my sexuality |
| Hope | I may have feared but I had hope |
| Pride | I swallowed my pride and participated in the trial |

To develop additional lyrics, the women split into groups, where they again stressed the themes of courage, hope, and control. One group wrote:[4]

There's always HOPE *nomangi sacrifiser* [even when I sacrifice]
Full of FEAR but i-*situation yangi iencouraga* [the situation gave me courage]
From bad to good *azange ngi luze ithemba* [I never lost hope]
Because I was in control
*Azange ngi luze* [I never lost] hope because I was in control

These two sets of lyrics powerfully illustrate the shared experiences of fear, hope, control, and sacrifice. Although women were initially scared to enroll in the trial and undergo HIV testing, they willingly gave themselves to the MDP301. Remaining hopeful through the trial process, participants were transformed into courageous individuals who gained command of their lives.

Narratives recounting the journey from fear to control through sacrifice and faith continued to be voiced in a subsequent segment of the workshop, when women were asked to tell their individual stories through lyrics. Like many other participants, Nombuyiso recalled having to overcome her fear of HIV testing: "I was asking myself many questions like 'what will happen if I find out that I'm positive?' I wanted to go and join [the trial] but I was afraid. Then I waited for about two months, having doubts." Her discovery that she was HIV negative was a "wake-up call . . . because it gave me an opportunity to check myself and take responsibility for my own health." In the following verse, Nombuyiso evoked these experiences:

*Ivari, iqiniso, that we are dying*
*But since ngazi istatus sam*
*Ngiye ngaqina isibindi, kwaphela Ukwesaba,*
*Kwavuka ithemba, nganqoba le doubt ngangena ihighway*
*Kwabamnandi ngazazi ncono*

It is the truth that we are dying
But since I know my status
I became strong, I was not afraid
My hope was resurrected
I overcame my fears and entered the highway
It was great and I knew myself better

Through these lyrics, Nombuyiso described testing HIV negative in the midst of the AIDS epidemic and going through her personal transformation. By the end of her involvement in the trial, she had emerged, knowledgeable of herself. The agent of change for Nombuyiso, as it was for many women, was HIV status. Being HIV negative gave Nombuyiso strength, confidence, and self-knowledge. Like others, she left the trial a believer.

Phetheni also wrote about the transformative effects of trial participation, recalling a Venda proverb about women possessing the courage and strength necessary to accomplish difficult tasks, such as holding hot objects. Referring to this proverb, Phetheni wrote:

*Kharivhonisane*
*Ndila ndi mupfa i athavha*
*Ahuna tshino fhatiwa nntha ha mazwifhi*
*Fhedzi thuthuwedzo rothe ri a i toda*
*Ngauri nga vhuthihi rido kunda*
*Mufumacadza u fara ludongo nga hufhisaho*
*Shangoni hodala rhuleme*
*Ndo dzhena icha mulingo fhedzi nda fhedza*
*Ndo bvelela uri ndi do kona uri huvena bvelaphandla*
*Do ima luhagala ngauri ndingo ndo ivona*
*Ro sikiwa i uri rivhe kundi*
*Nga lutendo lwanga na fulufelo langa udo vha na bvelelo dzwavhudi*
*Ri do upembela rido pembela*
*Uvhamufumakadzi u fanela uvhana tshivhindi*
*Nga dzhele ya vha fumakadza HIV ri do ivhulunga*
*Roguma uvha zwipondwa zwa HIV*


Let's show (help) each other
The path is thorny and it pierces
Nothing can be built on lies
All we need is courage
So that together we will conquer
The woman holds the hot clay pot
The world is full of hardships
I enrolled in the trials and I have finished
I have finished so that there can be progress
I stand tall talking about this study/trial

> We were born to be conquerors
> I hope that there will be good results
> Then we will rejoice
> To be a woman you must have courage
> With the gel for the women we will bury HIV
> Enough is enough to be victims of HIV

According to these lyrics, the MDP301 transformed women from hopeless, ignorant, and fearful people into courageous, hopeful, and brave subjects. Furthermore, the women's fortitude allowed them to endure the trial and develop a greater capacity for bearing the burden of suffering. Stressing women's inherent strength, Phetheni portrayed participants as conquerors who had escaped the bonds of victimhood.

For many participants, the catalysts for their transformation were sacrifice and faith. Women perceived their enrollment as a selfless act and acknowledged that they were willing to take risks in an effort to contribute to the testing and development of AIDS prevention technologies. Angry at rumors labeling the trial as harmful, a participant said, "People talk too much about the gel because it's not them using it. When they are testing the gel on us, it's what we want. It is true when they say we are taking risks—so what? I am proud of what I am doing because I want to see if this gel works so it can help many people. That is why at the end I tell myself that I am a lifesaver and I feel good about it." Participating in the trial was a personal sacrifice that women willingly undertook to help others. In her lyrics, Thabile described sacrificing herself for her family and friends. She wanted to assist in the fight against AIDS so that others could live. But through her sacrifice, Thabile had been given the strength to conquer obstacles that had previously stood in her way. Having faith in the outcome of her participation, Thabile is "waiting for a celebration to conquer all that comes against me." In her lyrics, Cora described a similar process:

> Uncertainty owing to my curiosity
> While fear was carefully covered and sealed for a glance
> The one was between courage and sacrifice
> That I had to blend the two and claim my pride
> From that moment I never looked back.

Thabile and Cora depicted themselves as surrendering their bodies, but they also noted that with sacrifice comes reward. On one hand, families, friends, and the community at large benefit through the development of new technologies to fight HIV. On the other, individuals gain through self-knowledge, control, and empowerment.

As with many of the other attitudes expressed by participants, the notion that women were sacrificing themselves through trial participation was not embraced by MDP301 staff. For one of the trial coordinators, the idea of sacrifice sent the "wrong message" because it implied that women were exposed to harm by their involvement. However, for participants, "sacrifice" drew from Christian narratives where faith and sacrifice led to redemption. Medicine, and particularly pharmaceuticals, expresses religious ideals and symbolism (Gordon 1988; van der Geest 2005). ARVs, for instance, have been compared to a sacrament for those with HIV (Comaroff and Comaroff 2011:188). Not only does medicine incorporate and reflect Christian ideals, churches themselves often embrace these meanings. Throughout southern Africa, AIDS has become intimately associated with morality and the church (Klaits 2010). It is not uncommon for churches to test members of their congregation for HIV and pray for the souls of those with AIDS. The religious connotations of medicine are especially meaningful in South Africa, where the adoption of Christianity, particularly African Zionism, appropriates Western messages and reformulates them within an African context (Comaroff 1985). In so doing, the hegemonic order is resisted through symbolism and ritual. Likewise, women's faith in their HIV status, coupled with their sacrifice for the MDP301, allows them to achieve biotechnical salvation. Adapting medical and moral significations of HIV, women create a new identity for themselves that affirms their own power and virtue.

Discussing their religious beliefs in interviews, women described praying for and seeking God's guidance throughout their participation in the MDP301. However, the song became a particular focus for Christian narratives. This was in part because of the important role that music played within the church context. Although the MDP301 decided to use *kwaito* music in an effort to reach a wide township audience, women commented that gospel would have been a more appropriate and popular style. While the MDP301 viewed the song as a way to spread information about the trial, for the women it was an expression of Christian ideals. After hearing the song on the radio, it was not uncommon for women to interpret it as sending a Christian message. In discussing the chorus, one woman said, "I think when they say *bambelela*, they are saying that you must hold on to God's word. I think God is the one who holds our lives. I can say when they say *bambelela*, it says focus on God's word because our lives depend on God. When you hold on to the word and pray, that is the only thing that can help." Participants had indeed drawn heavily from Christian narratives during the songwriting workshop. Lyrics of sacrifice and faith tied directly into religious beliefs. In describing her sacrifice, Thabile wrote:

> Praying to God that he must help me in each and every
> Uncertainty and give me courage to face my world
> And also improve my hope in taking care of those I love and cherish

The faith and courage women needed to become part of the MDP301 were directly linked to their Christian convictions. Sacrifice was a way through which the divine transformed potential danger into salvation.

As they discussed these perspectives with nonparticipants, women powerfully portrayed their trial experiences. At the songwriting workshop, the musicians were shocked and impressed by the fortitude of the women present. A few of the musicians, all male, had heard negative reports about the trial. Speaking to participants profoundly altered their perception of claims that the MDP301 was exploiting and injuring women. Through their stories, the women witnessed to the musicians and in a sense converted them. Drawing from Christian themes, Mandla commented:

> At first when they told me their stories I thought that these people are crazy. I was saying to myself, "How can you sacrifice your life like this?" Then I thought about in the Bible what Abraham did with his son Isaac, his only son. I thought that if you are a human being and living on this planet earth you don't have to be selfish. If you have a heart to offer something, then sacrifice, then do it because it is only God who knows your destination.

Reframing trial participation from senseless risk into sacred mission, Mandla commended the women for their extraordinary courage. This was echoed by several musicians, with a few describing participants as heroines. Not only

had these women sacrificed themselves for others, they had done so largely
without receiving any acclaim or reward. Sticks noted:

> I don't think those people get enough recognition because they risked
> their lives for this whole thing. I remember they used to talk about
> thinking whenever they were using this product and thinking that they
> are taking a risk and it could backfire in a really bad way. But they did
> it regardless, not thinking about themselves but thinking about the
> whole country and the whole world at large. Trying to prove that this gel
> can work or it couldn't. I remember there were a few people who were
> infected during the study. . . . They risked their lives and at the end of
> the day they didn't get anything in return. That is what I learned and I
> think they didn't even get enough recognition. Really, I respect them.

The musicians were so struck by the women's narratives that they composed
a verse honoring the participants' bravery and altruism:

> Thank our sisters for the living sacrifice that you did
> You give us hope in the moment of despair
> Sacrificed and risked to be in that study
> For all the homies
> Courage to be in control

Although this verse was not in the recorded version of the song, it pays
tribute to the women's experiences of sacrifice, hope, and ultimately control.

## SUCCESSFULLY DEMONSTRATING FAILURE

As the last trial participant formally exited the MDP301 in August 2009,
the clinics focused on organizing data files, reports, and documents for
analysis. All participants were told to return unused gel to the clinic,
and several home visits were undertaken to collect it, as all lots had to
be accounted for and incinerated. Meanwhile, the final data points were
submitted to the coordinating center in the United Kingdom. Despite the
closure of the 2 percent arm, there was excitement about the possibility of
success. After all, PRO 2000/5 had been proven to be effective, albeit not in
a statistically significant way, in the smaller HPTN 035 trial. Many of the

investigators and trial managers had that trial in mind, particularly because it had been so celebrated. Anna Forbes (2010), former deputy director of the GCM, recalls hearing about the HPTN 035 results: "Although premature, that rush of hope only reinforced my faith in the promise of microbicides. One South African trial site investigator emailed me that day to say trial participants at her site 'celebrated in true Zulu style' upon hearing the news that PRO 2000/5 might actually work. They were dancing." The long hours and hard work of many staff also encouraged them to have faith in the MDP301's success. This was particularly true of the site staff, who had spent month after month building and maintaining the infrastructure, recruiting volunteers, screening thousands of women, and following the lives of participants. For many, the trial had defined their working lives for almost five years.

The Johannesburg MDP301 staff learned the outcome of the trial on 19 November 2009, to prepare staff prior to the public announcement. The results had been surrounded by mystery and intrigue, as everyone analyzing them had been sworn to secrecy and signed nondisclosure agreements that warned of extreme penalties should they be broken. The Soweto and Orange Farm clinic nurses, doctors, and pharmacists gathered with the social science interviewers in the boardroom to hear the announcement. Most were optimistic, anticipating positive outcomes. We had chatted informally about the 2 percent arm closure, seeing it as an indication of the efficacy of the 0.5 percent arm; after all, wouldn't the IDMC have closed both arms if the 0.5 percent gel arm wasn't effective? Some staff filed silently into the boardroom, not daring to speak, offering only smiles and nods in greeting as they took their seats along the table.

The head of the clinical research division, tasked with divulging the results, gave nothing away, keeping a straight face. She began by asking the assembled researchers and clinicians what they thought the results were. Most voted in favor of efficacy—marginally so, but efficacy nonetheless. However, the MDP301 results were "flat," meaning that PRO 2000/5 had made no difference, even slightly, to HIV incidence among the trial participants. The good news was that the product had neither caused harm to those who used it nor increased their chances of acquiring HIV. But for many staff, the trial was seen to have failed, devaluing their personal investment in the study. One staff member said, "I am very disappointed about the results. I worked on this trial for so many years, hoping for a better result." For most of the clinic staff, who had come to know many of the participants, the outcome was deeply upsetting.

With the release of the results, many staff asked why the MDP301 produced different results from HPTN 035. In seeking to explain the failure of PRO 2000/5 in the MDP301, two popular explanations focused on a key methodology of clinical trial research: statistical probability. Trialists hypothesized that the HPTN 035 results were simply a result of chance and had no bearing whatsoever on predicting the efficacy of PRO 2000/5. In other words, despite rigorous randomization procedures, the study lacked the statistical power to demonstrate an effect. Yasmin Halima, director of the GCM, remarked in a press statement: "We all knew that the trend observed in HPTN 035 could have been due to chance" (Citizen News Service 2009). There was also a possibility that because MDP301 had been conducted at several different sites, contextual differences influenced the outcomes. However, the data analysis obfuscates these differences in an effort to reduce anomalies through the use of statistical models. Like many global health interventions, clinical trials are designed—and are therefore assumed to be implemented—in a uniform manner, and local cultural, social, and economic contexts are treated as "background static" (Adams et al. 2014:181). In other words, "local differences, and the specificities that local contexts reveal, often form a kind of black box in conventional approaches in global health, filled with variables that are regionally, culturally, and nationally different but not considered critical to the intervention or the research" (ibid.). Because local differences were not factored into the research design, variation could not be assessed. What may have worked at one site may not have at others, depending on adherence and the local epidemiology of HIV infections. Although Sir Austin Bradford Hill saw the use of statistical methods as inherently valuable, his model is increasingly unable to reconcile difference as trials are internationalized.

Once trial staff had been informed, the results were released to trial participants. It was early December, and trial administrators knew that many families would soon be leaving Johannesburg for home, so women were summoned to attend two hastily convened meetings at each clinic site.[5] To expedite the process, notifications were sent via text. The message read: "MDP301 trial results show that PRO 2000 gel is safe but does not reduce the risk of HIV transmission." For most, these texts came as a complete shock. In contrast to the lengthy process of screening and informed consent, the results were initially disseminated impersonally and without warning. Most importantly for participants, the gel was said to be ineffective. Upon hearing the results, one participant said simply, "We were sure that it prevented HIV." A few women suggested that the trial had calculated the results incorrectly, while others faulted their fellow participants. Blaming gel dumpers for a false result, one participant remarked, "I don't believe that the people used it the right way and that is why it didn't work. I think if they used it the right way, all of them, it would have worked."

Articulating questions and doubts regarding the accuracy of the results, many women refused to change their beliefs about the gel. Despite unambiguous trial messages to the contrary, participants continued to insist that it "did something." One woman declared that the doctors were simply wrong: because she did not contract HIV during her enrollment, it proved that the gel prevented infection. Others pointed to the gel's ability to cleanse their bodies, cure infections, and increase sexual pleasure: "The way we were using the gel it was like it was working because it has changed our sexual behavior. We thought you had made a mistake on the results." Participants' reliance on bodily cues to evaluate the gel was particularly evident during unblinding sessions, when they were informed of their assigned arm. Told that they had been using a placebo, some women immediately responded that they already knew. Those who reported no side effects assumed that they did not have gels containing PRO 2000/5. However, others engaged in strident arguments with the staff, asserting that because the gel had cleansed their bodies and prevented infections it could not have been a placebo. At these sessions, trial staff reiterated that the MDP301 records and results were accurate regardless of the experiences of the women. Yet even as trial coordinators attempted to convince participants to alter their views, AIDS activists remained committed to their belief in the effectiveness of microbicides.

Despite PRO 2000/5's lack of efficacy, medical researchers were quick to point out that the MDP301 was successful. In a sense, coordinators also asserted that the trial "did something." The MDP301 was regarded as an effective intervention in its own right for women's health, for African scientific capacity building, and for answering important scientific questions. First, it had used the gold standard of evidence-based medicine to generate a reliable result. The trial had performed its task efficiently and scientifically in line with *Good Clinical Practice* guidelines. Moreover, the product was safe to use. But many researchers and advocates also acknowledged that the achievements of the trial transcended scientific data. The MDP301 website notes that "even when a drug is found not to work, key lessons are learned which contribute to later successes" (MDP 2005). An official document on the trial results states that even though PRO 2000/5 was not effective in preventing HIV, the MDP301 "leaves a strong legacy. New laboratories have been equipped and accredited. Research center staff have gained experience and training in conducting clinical trials to the highest international standards. Many were supported to acquire degrees and diplomas which will advance their careers" (MDP 2009c). Its ability to benefit the communities involved led the MDP301 to be hailed as an achievement, particularly given that it was conducted in "developing countries" (Saxon 2012).

Perhaps the greatest outcome of the trial for advocates was the feeling that it had confirmed the ability of microbicides to impact women's lives positively. Acknowledging what many women told us, the trial reported that participants "have received counselling that will help them practice safe sex and lead healthier lives. They have a new understanding of their rights with respect to health care and know how to make the most of the care they receive. The trial has helped many women to discuss sex and HIV prevention options openly with their partners, and a surprising number report that their relationships have improved as a result" (MDP 2009b). MDP301 chair Sheena McCormack said, "Women reported that using it [PRO 2000/5] increased sexual pleasure and fostered intimacy by helping women talk about sex with their partners. So we know that we have the method right. Now we just need a product with the potency to stop HIV" (Citizen News Service 2009). On the MDP website, McCormack states unequivocally that the search for a microbicide has to continue, with "trials which are large enough to provide definitive evidence for whether or not a product works." MDP301 co-chair Jonathan Weber agrees: "It's still vital for us as scientists to continue to look for new ways of preventing HIV. There are many research groups exploring different avenues to tackle HIV; it is a slow process, but we are making progress. Now that we know this microbicide is not the answer, we can concentrate on other treatments that might be" (MDP 2009a). Responses such as this illustrate how a trial that some considered a failure can morph into a resounding success that robustly verifies the need for continued research and testing. It is the power of hope rather than effective chemicals that encourages investment and legitimizes the microbicide movement.

As trialists such as Weber and McCormack praised the positive outcomes of the MDP301, they failed to acknowledge the impermanence of these changes. Once the MDP301 closed its doors and women no longer had access to either the gel or medical testing, the transformations wrought by the trial disappeared. No longer able to use the gel as a cleansing agent, women also described experiencing period pain and vaginal problems. Asked to characterize their lives without the gel, focus group members replied,

*Respondent 1*: We are now suffering.

*Respondent 2*: We have infections again.

*Respondent 3*: The gel is no longer available and things are bad for me.

Other participants reported losing sexual enjoyment, while some added that intercourse was once again painful. Brenda said, "When it comes to sex with this gel, yes, I was feeling another king of enjoyment. So now condom alone, no, it is no longer that enjoyable. I am no longer lasting long. I used to last long with the gel. I am no longer even doing a different style." Without the pleasure of sex, relationships became strained. Tensions between partners were further exacerbated by the lack of HIV testing. Describing how her relationship with her husband had deteriorated, a participant commented, "During our participation in the study we had power because we knew where we stood. We were tested for HIV every three months but now if you ask your partner to do the HIV test he would say that he doesn't know what you are doing if you are not with him. The only thing that would happen now is blaming each other." Another noted that while she had been able to openly discuss sexual matters with her partner during the trial, she was now "back to square one." While male partners had been "treating us [participants] like queens," this was no longer the case: "It has gone back to the way that it was before." Observing that the trial had failed to engender long-lasting change, a participant declared, "That is why I also say that I am disappointed. I wish that the gel could come back."

Not only had the women lost access to the gel and HIV testing, but the strength, courage, and control they had gained on the trial evaporated. Although many participants clung to the belief that the gel worked, they nevertheless had to acknowledge that researchers and doctors disagreed with them. Knowing the gel would not be marketed, it seemed to the women as if their sacrifice had been for naught. Upset that PRO 2000/5 would not impact the lives of others, a participant said, "I felt sad, very much because I wanted these kinds of things to uplift other women. We would say 'we got this thing' but now that is all over." Having derived salvation from the gel's potential to effect profound transformation on a global level, participants could no longer have faith in a failed product. Brenda commented, "My heart was sore because I already told myself that when I got the gel I got the right thing. But when I heard that it wasn't working, I lost strength because the thing that was giving me strength was no longer working." Another participant noted, "I was very disappointed because I felt that . . . I don't have ammunition anymore. It was going to be something that belonged to me." Expressing defeat, a third participant added, "I was hoping that there was something that the women could hold on to." This statement is particularly poignant given that the MDP301 song urged women to "hold on." After the women learned the trial results, the lyrics became a reminder that the hope they were meant to embrace had vanished: "But now it is no longer there and we are left with the song only, what are we going to tell people?"

With the failure of PRO 2000/5, participants' claims to others that they were performing a noble task disappeared. Consequently, many participants had their strength replaced with vulnerability. Reflecting on his experiences during the songwriting workshop, a male musician said, "I am really disappointed that PRO 2000 wasn't successful because the ladies were so happy about it and they fell in love with it. They felt good about it. I think it was a close friend to the ladies and they felt safe." Yet, while the women's loss was remarked upon by those who knew them, microbicide advocates remained unaware that their empowerment had been temporary. This was in large part because trial coordinators failed to acknowledge that many of the changes had been the result of the MDP301's apparatus—HIV testing, education, and communal clinic waiting rooms—not PRO 2000/5. While the gel was generally praised by participants, it was also viewed as "a product on a shelf"—a commodity—whereas the trial was a process that positively impacted women's lives. Making the distinction between the gel and the trial, a participant said, "I do not think that I need a gel for empowerment, you know. I just needed it for protection whenever there was a mistake of maybe not using a condom. So I do not think I would need it for empowerment because I have empowerment through education." Crediting their personal transformations to the trial experience, many participants sought to continue in it. During information sessions about the trial results, former participants asked about other microbicide trials and how to enroll. While this caused some MDP301 staff to express concern that women were turning into "professional" participants to access cash payments, this was not the case. Women chose to join other trials to regain the illusive salvation they had achieved and lost through the MDP301. Rather than referring to these women as professionals, it would be more accurate to use the language of religion and say that they were following a calling.

# Conclusion

I n the years since the MDP301's December 2009 announcement, microbicides and their trials have changed considerably while nevertheless reproducing recurrent themes. Immediately after the MDP301 results were released, it seemed as if the allure of microbicides was coming to an end. That same year, the Alliance for Microbicide Development, a vital lobbyist for research funding, closed its doors. The alarms had begun sounding a couple of years earlier: John Moore, an immunologist at Weill Cornell Medical College in New York, had declared, "The microbicide field is drinking in the last-chance saloon. If it has many more problems, it's finished" (quoted in Check 2007:110). Others had agreed that the situation was desperate. McGill University virologist Mark Wainberg had stated that microbicides "cannot afford to take a further hit" (ibid.). Indeed, repeated product failures increasingly impacted microbicide advocacy. Concerned that poor trial results could lead to the abandonment of microbicides, Polly Harrison (2011) noted that "we have not regrouped as a dedicated constituency. Some think the field has matured to the point where specific microbicide advocacy is no longer required. I disagree; much organized conversation and advocacy remain essential. The final lessons for advocacy for microbicides and women's particular needs have not yet been told."

Despite repeated setbacks, microbicide supporters continued to follow a familiar pattern of linking activism, women's rights, and hope. Amid calls for further research, the third generation of microbicides was developed and tested. As polyanion inhibitors such as PRO 2000/5 were abandoned, researchers turned their attention to proven HIV treatments, notably antiretrovirals (ARVs). Unlike previous microbicides, the new generation was founded on an established body of evidence that demonstrated the therapeutic effectiveness of ARVs in treating AIDS and lowering viral loads. The same drugs that transformed the wasted bodies of AIDS sufferers into healthy survivors were now placed within vaginal gels to target viral replication directly (Lederman et al. 2006). Advocates once again expressed optimism that an efficacious microbicide would be identified and marketed quickly. Yet, regardless of these innovations, microbicides remain more valuable as an idea than a reality.

## SUSTAINING THE ECONOMY OF HOPE

As more aggressive pharmaceutical agents than surfactants, ARV-based microbicides seemed far more certain to yield results (Omar and Bergeron 2011). The first major trial of this third generation of microbicides tested a gel containing 1 percent tenofovir. Funded by USAID and run by Centre for the AIDS Program of Research in South Africa, the CAPRISA 004 trial lasted for over 30 months and involved 889 women. The results showed partial protection of 39 percent overall, but higher rates of protection were recorded among women who used the gel more frequently (Karim et al. 2010). The results received an unprecedented standing ovation at the International AIDS Conference in Rome and seemed to confirm a long-standing assumption among researchers, that routine adherence was the most important factor in demonstrating efficacy (Mansoor et al. 2014).

Like other advocates who had struggled for years, Polly Harrison (2011) felt vindicated for believing that a microbicide could prevent HIV: "I'm thrilled! Now we can say that topical microbicides have an accepted identity as an HIV prevention technology worth pursuing. We've had some long dark years sprinkled with disappointment, some loss of faith and, frankly, some disdain. To see the joy and hope in so many quarters is beyond gratifying." At a consultative meeting held in Johannesburg in 2010, convened by the South African National AIDS Council, the Wits Reproductive Health and HIV Institute, and the Treatment Action Campaign, a South African AIDS treatment lobby group, most of the participants called for the immediate availability of the gel. As Helen Rees from the WRHI remarked, "The discomfort we all have is that if this [product] is working, shouldn't we be pushing its use as quickly as possible?" (IRIN 2010). This view was also voiced by Zena Stein, who commented that the gel was "both safe enough and effective enough to be made immediately available, under controlled conditions, to women in high risk populations." She added, "One must bear in mind that every woman who does become infected will in time require treatment for the rest of her life. Prevention is not only humane; it is also sensible health policy" (Stein and Susser 2010). But, despite these endorsements, a tenofovir microbicide would not be released to the public.

While microbicide activists celebrated, regulatory authorities and scientists felt that the trial had provided insufficient evidence for licensure, arguing that more placebo-controlled trials were needed for a topical microbicide to be identified (Haire et al. 2012). The trial was regarded as only a "proof of concept." While researchers primarily employed bioethical arguments to justify the decision not to go to market, it was also a financial one. Licensure of tenofovir gel would have had major implications for the field of experimental microbicide research. The gel would have been transformed from an experimental product to a "standard of care" pharmaceutical, meaning it would have to be included in any future trial of a new microbicide. This would have increased not only the complexity of testing similar drugs in subsequent clinical trials but also the cost (ibid.). Ensuing microbicide trials would attract less attention, and the economy of hope, which has been invested in for years, would be put at risk.

In response to calls for additional assessment, a confirmatory trial was planned. Toward the end of 2010, FDA representatives met with CONRAD, the US-based trial sponsor, manufacturer, and supplier of tenofovir, and agreed to conduct another, larger trial to confirm CAPRISA's results.[1] Named Vaginal and Oral Interventions to Curb the Epidemic (VOICE), the trial was run by the University of Pittsburgh–based Microbicide Trials Network (MTN) and funded by the NIH. Enrolling 5,029 women in Uganda, South Africa, and Zimbabwe, VOICE would not only reevaluate a 1 percent tenofovir gel, but also evaluate tablets containing the drug. Although pills were being tested, researchers anticipated that a topical microbicide delivered to the vaginal mucosa—the site of exposure to HIV—would be safer and more effective than a systemically absorbed drug in tablet form. Yet in September 2011, the VOICE data safety monitoring board (DSMB) recommended that the gel arm be halted for reasons of futility.[2] Then two months later, the DSMB made the same recommendation for the tenofovir tablet arm. When the results were tabulated, the VOICE researchers reported no reduction in HIV incidence with any of the tested interventions (Marrazzo et al. 2015). In contrast to the celebrations that greeted the results of CAPRISA, researchers mourned the trial at a MTN meeting in Cape Town by observing a moment of silence and distributing cupcakes with purple and green frosting—the MTN colors.

The results of the VOICE trial were described as "perplexing" (van der Straten et al. 2012), particularly in the light of CAPRISA's success. As explanations were sought, it was revealed that poor adherence to the drug was the main reason for its inability to show effect. An analysis of pharmacokinetic values in blood samples taken during VOICE led researchers to conclude that less than 30 percent of participants had used either the gel or the tablets (Marrazzo et al. 2015). This came as a complete surprise, as throughout the trial the vast majority of women had reported almost perfect compliance.[3] Such large-scale and widespread nonadherence was unanticipated and unprecedented, leading to extensive press coverage. The online service *e-Health News* declared, "Africa: Big Prevention Blow as Women Reject One-a-Day ARV" (Thom 2013). The *Weekly Mail and Guardian* newspaper headline read, "Women Confound HIV Researchers" (8 March 2013). *Science* led with "Human Nature Sinks HIV Prevention Trial" (Cohen 2013). Reports of low adherence led many researchers to distrust and dismiss the accounts of participants as fiction and lies. As a South African HIV scientist put it, participants had "hoodwinked" the trial. As a discourse of deceitful participants grew, researchers raised questions about women's behavior and their reasons for wanting to participate in clinical trials.

While microbicide trialists sought to enroll members of the population they considered most vulnerable to HIV infection—impoverished African women—they simultaneously regarded these participants as unreliable. The structural inequalities in African communities were thought to drive women to trials, attracted by the resources on offer. In a context of poverty and limited health infrastructure, continued access to health screening and treatment was often as important as cash remuneration (Delany-Moretlwe, Stadler et al. 2011). A social scientist commented about the VOICE trial results:

> A lot of folks in really resource-limited settings might quite sensibly say, "Well, I could get money for participating in this trial, and I'd get a lot of health benefits—monitoring of my health and wellness, good counseling, access to condoms—so it's a good deal. I have no intention of taking the pill, but I'm not going to *say* that." (Auerbach 2013)

In attempting to escape poverty and improve their health, women were blamed for their behavior. A clear distinction was made between altruistic and selfish motivations. Whereas "altruism is crucial for patients to become good, compliant subjects in a clinical trial" (Fisher 2008:89), the "professional participant" or "veteran" knows how to work the system by participating repeatedly in trials for their own benefit (Tishler and Bartholomae 2003).

Selfish participants were blamed not only for poor trial outcomes but also for potentially prolonging the AIDS pandemic and suffering of others. Reflecting on the VOICE results, IRMA chair Jim Pickett (2013) wrote, "I think it is unfair to everyone, especially highly impacted communities where HIV rates are soaring, and where the crisis is anything but over, for trial participants to sign informed consents and derive individual benefits from trials without fully engaging in the study protocols that would allow for potential population benefits." Statements such as this chastise nonadherent participants, portraying them as immoral. Interestingly, narratives of greedy women seeking to cheat the trial mirror those of MDP301 participants regarding gel dumpers. Whether clinical trials are understood from the perspective of participants or medical researchers, they are projects that establish a moral order. MDP301 participants would agree with researchers' statements stressing the importance of altruism when enrolling in trials. In fact, the selflessness associated with honest trial participation was one of the factors that allowed women to assert their morality not only inside but also outside of a medical context. Even as researchers become more inclined to cast participants as irresponsible, participants themselves can reframe this discourse to highlight their own exceptional commitment to helping others.

As blame for lack of efficacy shifted from chemistry to behavior, participants have come under increasing scrutiny. Growing mistrust has led to the development of new methods of interrogating women's bodies to assess adherence. Wary of relying on interviews, trial coordinators have turned to computer-aided methods, blood tests, and gel applicator screenings. Computer-aided self-interviews, which participants complete in isolation, are being administered in more trials in an effort to remove bias resulting from the presence of a human interviewer (Minnis et al. 2009; Pool et al. 2010). In other cases, visual inspections of vaginal applicators using ambient and ultraviolet lighting to detect vaginal secretions are utilized to monitor compliance (Moench et al. 2012). The Population Council has begun distributing vaginal applicators that change color after insertion (Wallace et al. 2007) as well as employing so-called smart applicators that use biometric tags, and "wise bags" with SMS technology that send messages to a computer each time they are opened (van der Straten et al. 2013). While microbicides are intended to give women control over their bodies, these new investigative apparatuses do just the opposite. This contradiction has been lost on most researchers, who consider medical surveillance necessary for a positive trial outcome. Female empowerment through microbicides is therefore to be achieved, ironically, by subjecting women's bodies to ever more stringent monitoring.

## THE ANTHROPOLOGISTS AT THE BACK OF THE ROOM

As they attempt to explain why so many women were not using their gels, medical researchers have continued to invoke the social and the cultural (Geary and Bukusi 2014). As a result, microbicide researchers increasingly solicit the work of social scientists to better understand the motivations and experiences of trial participants. For decades, anthropology has debated how best to engage with the medical profession (Cassell 2002; Hemmings 2005; Shand 2005; Singer and Baer 1995). Some argue that participating in a medical context, such as clinical trials, transforms anthropologists into handmaidens of biomedical hegemony, while others believe that only through a meaningful engagement with the medical profession will we be able to effect positive change in clinical protocols and procedures. However, the reality is far from this simple dichotomy. As a part of a larger team, the work of social scientists is constrained by the conventions of clinical research. While social scientists play a consultative role in most contemporary microbicide trials, the mixed methods approach of the MDP301 has yet to be replicated. In recent trials, social science researchers have been restricted to asking set questions to a small number of participants and have been prohibited from engaging in participant observation, as well as forbidden to visit or speak with participants outside of the confines of the clinic.

Despite the awareness of and interest in social scientific contributions toward clinical trial research, some scientists have expressed concerns about the validity and morality of ethnographic approaches. First, anthropological case studies and observations are frequently discounted as "soft" observational findings, which are labeled "anecdotal" when compared to "hard" data. With the current reliance on statistics, quantitative figures are required for funding, testing, and licensure. In this context, less easily enumerated textual accounts of AIDS are "set aside as perhaps interesting, but largely irrelevant when it comes to policy" (Allen 2006). Consequently, trialists often cast social scientists, and anthropologists in particular, as contributing a perspective that fails to aggressively advance the goals of medical research. Second, qualitative methodologies, particularly participant observation, are viewed as potentially unethical. Whereas a clinical setting reminds participants that they are engaging in medical research, bioethicists worry that people talking to researchers on the street or in a pool hall will be unaware of their participation or unable to decline. Portrayed as a clandestine activity, participant observation is thought to fall outside of the conventions of methods that are regulated through informed consent procedures (Fassin 2006). For example, attempts to record conversations in the waiting room of one clinical trial resulted in protocol violations being issued by the study sponsor.

Although anthropologists are increasingly incorporated into clinical trial research, they are simultaneously being excluded from it. To illustrate the ways in which this tension between incorporation and exclusion is played out in everyday institutional settings, we turn to a meeting we attended at the NIH headquarters in Bethesda, Maryland, at the end of 2014. Facilitated by the MTN, the meeting was intended to address growing concerns about young women, their personal risk of infection, and their apparent lack of interest in stopping the spread of HIV. In theory, the organizers sought to better understand sexual decision-making in African women and their use of HIV prevention products. The backdrop to the meeting was the assumption that health experts were not sure what women, especially young women, really wanted or needed. The MTN sought to engage more broadly with social and behavioral scientists to explore contextual factors such as culture, economics, politics, and media that impact women's lives. Present at the meeting were investigators and staff from the African sites of the MTN studies, sociologists who had worked in African settings on adolescent sexuality, public health researchers from affiliated organizations, and representatives of a pan-African study on using a television drama to promote behavior change among adolescents.

The first item on the agenda featured the stories of young women at various MTN sites across Africa. Prior to the meeting, staff at these sites had been instructed to collect accounts of those who had experienced difficulties when making sexual choices and negotiating sex with men. As these vignettes were presented, a common theme was often repeated: Young women had trouble insisting on condom use and were worried that their partners could be infecting them with HIV. In each tale, the subject was cast as poor, socially constrained, and vulnerable. But each of these women expressed a strong desire to be protected from HIV, as well as to achieve greater levels of social and economic freedom. At the end of the session, several attendees commented on the close degree of similarity among the stories, noting that they reinforced what microbicide advocates had been saying for years: African women are vulnerable, but this situation could be ended through effective HIV prevention. However, the concurrence of these narratives was not surprising, given that each staff member received specific instructions regarding the theme and content of the stories they were to collect. Rather than portraying the complexity of women's experiences, this exercise produced a homogenized and simplified rendering in keeping with the beliefs of microbicide advocates. As in other development discourse, history and politics were ignored to construct a uniquely solvable problem that aid organizations are exclusively able to address (Ferguson 1990).

The primary session of the meeting consisted of research presentations, during which participants discussed their findings and highlighted areas in which further investigation was necessary. Reflecting public health's preoccupation with the role of culture in health behavior, the organizers asked us to speak on the barriers that African beliefs could create in clinical trial participation. Other individuals reviewed equally general topics, such as partners, stigma, family, and peers. Toward the end of the session, a consensus emerged, with the majority of attendees agreeing that researchers possessed a relatively small amount of information on young women's attitudes and behavior regarding sex. One area of particular note was vaginal insertion practices. Commenting that an extensive survey had yet to be conducted, meeting participants asked one another what substances women were using and speculated about the frequency and distribution of these practices. Another topic deemed worthy of further study was women's interpretation of microbicide gels. How did they understand the gel? What did they think it was doing in their bodies? Why were some women using it and others not?

Attempting to answer some of these questions, we reviewed our own work as well as the extensive literature on the social meaning of pharmaceuticals and clinical trials. We suggested that flow was a central theme in women's understanding of the gel and its ability to effect change in their bodies. Revisiting our data on the use of drying agents, we contended that experiences of painful sex often impinged on idealized accounts of dry sex. Noting that the gel could also be invoked in narratives of pleasure and personhood, we argued that microbicides have become incorporated into existing ontologies. Therefore, women's participation in trials was about much more than seeking remuneration or health care. Clinical trials allowed women to renegotiate social relationships tactically and in the process construct an empowered identity. As we spoke, several people nodded their heads and commented that our research did touch on many of the issues we were discussing. However, few people saw our research as being helpful. We were told that while we could recount interesting stories about women on the MDP301, our research was merely anecdotal, not factual. "Hard data," quantitative data, was needed before any true conclusions could be drawn. While our perspectives on culture and its potential danger were solicited, we were largely excluded from conversations about behaviors considered to be measurable.

On the final day of the meeting, participants were split up into groups, to produce lists of critical research questions for shaping future clinical trials. We were assigned to a group tasked with examining the cultural challenges young women face in adopting effective HIV prevention technologies. The group referred to as "Cultural Factors" comprised three anthropologists, a sociologist, an epidemiologist from a contract research organization, and a facilitator from the NIH. As in our previous presentations, we argued that culture was complex and that there was no such thing as a single "African culture." The other members of our group strongly disagreed with us, insisting that in fact young African women were largely the same across the continent. Seeking to shift the focus of the discussion, we then advocated a move away from an exclusively culture-based model to one that also acknowledged the economic and political. The NIH participant objected, noting that clinical trials were not political enterprises. Reminding her that the NIH and the trials it conducted were funded by the US government, we asserted that politics were in fact central to the international medical project. She countered that while this might be the case, openly acknowledging this would potentially result in even more rumors of harm circulating around trial sites and discourage women from enrolling. Frustrated at our interjections, one participant told us, "For people who claim to want to listen to others, you sure do talk a lot."

As we presented our discussion to the meeting, it elicited a great deal of feedback from the audience. When our representative began by announcing that we could at least agree that culture existed, everyone erupted in applause. However, the statement that our group felt we were asking the wrong question by focusing only on culture was greeted with a collective groan. While the audience widely agreed that social science input was important, one person commented that this research should be conducted by investigators who would not question or critique the underlying assumptions of clinical trials. Instead of redesigning protocols or suggesting new paradigms, the role of social science, we were told, should be to support existing endeavors. A participant commented that he was glad not to have been a member of our discussion group. Anthropologists, he said, always had to complicate matters and question the question. All the NIH and other health organizations wanted, we were informed, was a list of bullet points that mirrored their priorities. Why, he asked, couldn't we just give them what they wanted? Our answer was that people's lives are complex and cannot be reduced to a series of bullet points. By the time the meeting concluded, many of the other participants were referring to us as "the anthropologists at the back of the room." While this label ostensibly alluded to our choice of seats, it also seemed to capture our status as peripheral participants in the global health project.

Even though anthropological research within clinical trials might be regarded as marginal by some, we believe that this work is important. Clinical trials are not only scientific, medical, and economic projects; they are also social and political ventures. As the number of international trials continues to increase, more people will have their worlds impacted by these endeavors. But while biomedicine's footprint is expanding, it is not occurring in the way anticipated by trialists and pharmaceutical advocates. The outcomes of medical research are far more profound than data regarding "efficacy" or "acceptability" would suggest. Trials have social and experiential lives that are engendered by the research process itself and transcend clinical narratives and quantitative figures. In exposing people to experimental drugs that are inherently uncertain, clinical trials encourage participants to appropriate medical discourses for their own ends. Although testing a new pharmaceutical is risky and requires participants to submit their bodies to surveillance, it also transforms these same participants from passive objects to agentive subjects as *materia medica* is situated within embodied everyday contexts. As women on the MDP301 said, the gel was good for a great many things. In the future, those who participate in the research process will no doubt continue to do so in innovative and surprising ways.

# Appendix

## BAMBELELA

### Intro

Microbicides, microbicides,
    microbicides.

Microbicides, microbicides,
    microbicides.

### Chorus A

Bambelela, bambelela, qinisela.
Bambelela, bambelela, qinisela.

Hold on, hold on, hold on tight.
Hold on, hold on, hold on tight.

### Verse 1

Ba chele s'koko, yes.
Wo! Phola u-relaxe guluva.
Aba kasi khombisivikela igciwane
Kodwa bamba isandla sam s
    weetie ungasabi.
Ngikusikele, ngikubekele
    nga le microbicide.
Eqondane ngqo na labo abazitika
    ngoko cantsi
Kodwa abanganalo igciwane
    lekagawulayo.
Uzocwaningisiswa kahle ukuthi
    ingasithiba na izifo socantsi.
Eish! Kodwa abancelisayo,
Hai kabe one side,
Hai kabe one side.

Tell them boss, yes.
Wait! Relax, relax, my thug [friend].
They haven't yet proven that it can
    prevent HIV
But hold my hand, my sweetheart,
    don't be afraid.
Let me tell you, let me tell you about
    this microbicide.
It is aimed at those who are
    sexually active
But not those who are infected
    with HIV.
It is being researched to see if it can
    prevent STIs.
Oh! But those who are breastfeeding,
Sorry you are excluded,
Sorry you are excluded.

## Chorus B

Bambelela, bambelela, qinisela.
Bambelela, bambelela, qinisela.
Ngithi bambelela, qinisela.

Hold on, hold on, hold on tight.
Hold on, hold on, hold on tight.
I say hold on, hold on tight.

## Verse 2

Hola dee, wa ithola daideng?
Ka nako ye o keke wabe wa ithola
PRO 2-Stena ntwana! Eish!
It's still on trial ntwana! Au!
Ngebezwa ba kuluma ngayo,
Ba thetha ngayo, ba bua ka yona.
Ka nako ye ntwana, o keke wabe
    wa ithola.

Hello there, do you get that thing?
This time you won't get it
PRO 2-brick boy! Oh!
It's still on trial, boy! Oh!
I heard them talking about it,
They talk about it, they talk about it,
At this time, boy, you won't get it.

## (repeat Chorus A)

## Verse 3

Cathula nathi umungana ncelisi. (Auu!)
Cathula nathi umungana igciwane. (Ai!
    Ai!)
Umu ufuni ku boni imiphumela nje
    nga kwaMakhanya.
Kwaze kwa bakhanyela, ba phuma
    ebumnyameni.
Ungathi ngiya bona emhleni yonkana.
Se ngi lala phansi, ngi vuke phezulu
Nga lebomnandi be gele ngo mashesha
Wa thela wa yekha umngani
    we condomu.
Cha mana we bhuti, one gel,
    one round
Phezu kwe condomu.
Ozubuzwa, ubunandi, obulapho.

Walk with us if you are not
    breastfeeding. (Ohh!)
Walk with us if you do not have the
    disease [HIV]. (Hey! Hey!)
If you want the results, like the
    Makhanyas.
Finally they got the light, they got out
    of darkness.
I wish I could see each day.
When I sleep below and wake up
    on top
With this enjoyment from the gel it
    comes quickly
Moving freely without fear, a friend to
    the condom.
No, wait, my brother, one gel,
    one round
As well as the condom.
You will feel that enjoyment there.

## (repeat Chorus B)

## Verse 4

Ahe! PRO 2000
Endla rirhandzu, ringeta ku
    kunghuhata
Xivatlanamindzeko, ndzi katsa na jazi
    ra tatana
Mapfuneta swa vutomi,
Jazi ra tatana ra pfuneta swa vutomi.
Ahe! Ahe! Ahiyeni.

(repeat Chorus A)

Hello! PRO 2000
Make love, try to prevent
The thing that is killing the nation
    [HIV], use the condom
The helper of lives,
The condom saves lives.
Hello! Hello! Let's go.

# Notes

## INTRODUCTION

1. Formal interviews and group discussions were audio recorded, transcribed, and when necessary translated into English by MDP301 social science staff. Our informants mainly spoke either isiZulu or seSotho.
2. Of the 2,508 women enrolled at the Johannesburg site, 150 were randomly selected by an external statistician to participate in serial in-depth interviews (IDIs), at clinic visit weeks 4, 24, and 52. In addition, trial women who were not selected for interviews were invited to take part in 25 focus group discussions. Community members who were not involved in the trial participated in 19 focus groups. On average each focus group comprised 8 participants.
3. Six women said that their partners disliked the gel, and the remaining five reported unwanted symptoms, reduced sexual enjoyment, and inconvenience.

## CHAPTER 1

1. Research among diaphragm users in Kenya did, however, highlight the advantages of having a secret method to use that their partners could not detect (Okal et al. 2008).
2. The commentary on drunk clients was recorded during the 2003 Reproductive Health Priorities Conference, Johannesburg, South Africa, 14–17 October.
3. During the Soccer World Cup held in South Africa in 2010, the Rape-aXe achieved some popularity in the media, largely fueled by a moral panic of football hooliganism.
4. Epidemiological modeling studies critiqued the notion of microbicides affecting condom use and presented counterevidence (Foss et al. 2003).
5. This tension between the structural and the biomedical has not disappeared and is part of an ongoing debate in discussions about the role of biomedical research and social determinants of HIV infection (Bell 2003; Roberts and Matthews 2012).

CHAPTER 2

1.  It had been initially determined that 1 percent tenofovir gel applied before and after vaginal intercourse was 39 percent effective in reducing HIV acquisition, with a trend toward 54 percent effectiveness in the most adherent women (Karim et al. 2010). However, the same gel applied daily was ineffective in a subsequent trial (Marrazzo et al. 2015).

2.  As a response to the short-course AZT trial, the Helsinki Declaration was revised for the sixth time and guidelines were put in place to ensure that a placebo would not be used if treatment standards had already been determined (Petryna 2005:188).

3.  The Belgian study, funded by WHO, had important consequences for future microbicide safety studies, standardizing the use of colposcopy to assess safety (Van Damme 2004).

4.  Years later, another study showed that N-9 gel resulted in increasing "levels of inflammatory cytokines, which would activate potential host cells for HIV" (Ravel et al. 2012).

5.  Carraguard itself was sourced from the US chemicals company FMC Technologies.

6.  The statistical insignificance of the results was potentially due to poor adherence to the product by trial participants (Ramjee et al. 2010).

7.  According to researchers from the Microbicides Development Programme, Hlongwa employed deception and subterfuge to gain access to a trial participant in a different trial—the MDP301—by posing as an official with the health department (Robinson et al. 2010).

8.  Of the nine-thousand-plus women who completed the trial, more than five thousand were referred for treatment, care, and support.

9.  In 2002, Clare Short, UK secretary of state for international development, endorsed microbicides as a gender and equity issue and donated £14 million to the British Medical Research Council, Imperial College, and 5 African countries (Boseley 2009).

10. In January 2009, Endo Pharmaceuticals—a US-based company specializing in marketing pain medication—purchased Indevus. Although the understanding between Indevus and the MDP301 was supposed to be sustained in the takeover, toward the end of 2009 this appeared to be uncertain (WHO 2010).

11. Women were not eligible if they were unable or unwilling to provide a reliable method of contact, were likely to move out of the area within 12 months, were likely to have sex more than 14 times a week on a regular basis (a regulatory requirement was that no more than 60 applicators were to be dispensed every 4 weeks), used spermicides regularly, were pregnant or within 6 weeks

postpartum, had a severe clinical or laboratory abnormality, needed referral for assessment of a suspicious cervical lesion, had received treatment to the cervix or other gynecological procedure within 30 days of enrollment, were allergic to latex, or were participating or had participated in another clinical trial that was likely to affect the primary efficacy endpoint within 30 days before enrollment.

12. The face-to-face meetings usually ended with a celebration, with researchers dancing and on occasion singing "MDP" to the tune of "YMCA."

## CHAPTER 3

1. Students made up 12 percent of respondents, and 1 percent did not reveal their employment status.

2. Because rumors are inherently fluid, it was difficult to quantify the number of people who either firmly supported or firmly disagreed with them. But we can assert that the majority of Sowetans and Orange Farmers were aware of tales that cast the trial as existentially exploitative and in some cases as a disguise for genocide.

3. Ironically, it is malls like Maponya that have all but killed off the small convenience shops, known as *spazas*, that operate from roadside stalls and from residential homes. The malls thus deprive households of vital incomes.

4. The estimated value of tourism generated by Soweto is R85 million ($8.5 million), and 70,000 tourists visit the township annually (Krige 2011:129).

5. Soweto had an average of 24 people per housing plot (Crankshaw and Hart 1990). While about half of the one-room structures erected in Soweto's backyards accommodated two people, 23 percent had four or more in the single room (Crankshaw et al. 2000).

6. The child support grant is a state welfare payment of R250 ($25) per month per child under the age of 18, to caregivers who individually earn less than R30,000 ($3,000) per year or have an annual combined income of less than R60,000 ($6,000).

7. A survey of antenatal clinic attendees in Soweto notes that 21 percent of women who reported transactional sex were more likely to test positive for HIV and experience partner violence (Dunkle et al. 2004b).

8. Sexual violence is also strongly linked to HIV spread; one survey reports that 25 percent of women have a lifetime prevalence of sexual violence (Jewkes et al. 2003). In 1996, a survey conducted in Johannesburg found that 67 percent of all respondents were victims of crime, while 37 percent were victims more than once (Ashforth 2005:36). Engagement in crime functioned as a rite of passage into adulthood for some men (Glaser 2000).

9. The uprisings of the mid- to late 1980s that impacted Soweto, Sebokeng, and Evaton also resulted in refugees seeking less turbulent locations such as Orange Farm (Sapire 1992), while a few (less than 20 percent) originated from the former Bantustans, located far from Johannesburg (Crankshaw and Hart 1990).

10. In future sessions, trial staff answered these questions by asserting the following: "(1) If condoms are used correctly, they are effective and not dangerous. (2) We ask women to record when they use condoms and when they do not. Data to determine the efficacy of PRO 2000/5 will be culled from instances when women did not use condoms. (3) Women who test HIV positive will be given support and referred to public health ART distribution centers."

11. While we have no quantitative figures, we believe that women who concealed gel use from their partners were in the minority.

12. White (2000:18) notes that blood-selling rumors in East and Central Africa were derived from witchcraft beliefs.

13. Similar accusations were uncovered in Zambia, where rumors of the MDP301 trial's association with Satanism were far more common.

## CHAPTER 4

1. It should be noted that the desire for a dry and tight vagina is not confined to sub-Saharan Africa. In Western countries a similar ideal exists and can be witnessed in the many products and medical procedures that women undergo to "perfect" their vaginas (Braun and Kitzinger 2001).

2. Women most often used the English word "dry" or the isiZulu equivalent, *wu omisa*.

3. Women recorded precoital and postcoital intravaginal cleaning and insertions in their coital diaries and were also asked about their everyday routines during clinical and social science interviews.

4. The symbolic association between ancestors, sex, and snuff motivates these beliefs and practices (Murray 1975).

5. Drying and tightening agents were just one form of body practice that was used to improve the sensation of sex in an effort to retain partners. From the age of approximately fifteen, some young women were instructed to stretch their labia minora to form "curtains" that were reputed to grip a man's penis and ensure his devotion. Women could also insert *muthi* vaginally to please and control a man magically.

6. In the KwaZulu-Natal site of the MDP301, 7 of 63 interviewed participants reported inserting substances vaginally to enhance sexual experiences (Gafos et al. 2010:932).

7. The KwaZulu-Natal arm of the trial reported similar results, with 49 of 63 women and 4 of 8 men asserting that the gel enhanced their sexual pleasure (Gafos et al. 2010:935).

## CHAPTER 5

1. To determine if the gel was in fact the source of these symptoms, participants engaged in a number of activities, including consulting the clinic, stopping gel use, and continuing with the gel while more closely monitoring bodily changes.
2. *Ukungcolo* (isiZulu) and *ditshila* (seSotho) have been translated as "dirt."
3. Other women used blotting paper to soak up and remove excess fluid from the vagina.
4. A phase I study of PRO 2000/5 showed that a 4 percent concentration did produce higher rates of epithelial adverse events than lower dosages (Van Damme et al. 2000).
5. There is no evidence to suggest that women who asserted that they were given the placebo used it less frequently when having intercourse than those who believed that they were given an active gel.
6. Participants in another microbicide trial also reported thinking that the placebo would be watery (FHI 2008).
7. Out of an enrollment of approximately 1,800 women, 229 pregnancies were reported.
8. Despite suffering from heavy discharge, Andiswa did not consult a public health care clinic because she "was scared of the bad treatment I would get because they become very rude if you are suffering from a sexually related sickness. I was trying to avoid that."

## CHAPTER 6

1. When informed by phone that they were on the discontinued arm, a number of women stated that they already knew they were using the 2 percent gel because of the side effects they were experiencing.
2. While those participants reporting multiple sexual partners were most at risk for contracting HIV during their enrollment, so too were younger women (18–24 years; Delany-Moretlwe, Nanoo, et al. 2011). Once a participant tested HIV positive, the MDP301 facilitated their entry into a treatment program. Some participants asserted that the women who became HIV positive on the trial did so because they were not using the gel as directed.
3. The complete lyrics for the final version are available in the Appendix.

4. Lyrics are reproduced here in the language or languages chosen by each woman. Translations follow the lyrics not originally written in English.

5. As predicted, the meetings were poorly attended: of the 448 participants who confirmed plans to be at the meetings, only 177 (39.51 percent) actually appeared (Saxon 2012). A similarly low rate also occurred during the unblinding process. Of 412 participants who were contacted, only 46 came to the clinic to learn of their assigned trial arm.

## CONCLUSION

1. Gilead Sciences, a biopharmaceutical corporation, granted the license to CONRAD to develop and manufacture tenofovir, and, if it was proven efficacious, to arrange for its distribution in resource-limited countries as a microbicide.

2. Futility outcomes mean that the trial is unlikely to be able to show any effect of the product being tested, even if it were to continue. It does not mean, however, that the product is ineffective.

3. Despite relying exclusively on self-reporting, we believe that there was a higher level of adherence during the MDP301 precisely because the explicit link between sex and insertion of a vaginal gel dovetailed neatly with women's ideas of flow and of sexual pleasure. In contrast, the daily dose required in VOICE was separated from the act of sex and consequently any meaningful association was lost.

# References

Abaasa, Andrew, Angela Crook, Mitzy Gafos, Zacchaeus Anywaine,
Jonathan Levin, Symon Wandiembe, Ananta Nanoo et al.
   2013 "Long-Term Consistent Use of a Vaginal Microbicide Gel among HIV-1
      Sero-Discordant Couples in a Phase III Clinical Trial (MDP 301) in Rural
      South-West Uganda." *Trials* 14.
Abadie, Roberto
   2010 *The Professional Guinea Pig: Big Pharma and the Risky World of Human
      Subjects.* Durham, NC: Duke University Press.
Adams, Vincanne, Nancy J. Burke, and Ian Whitmarsh
   2014 "Slow Research: Thoughts for a Movement in Global Health." *Medical
      Anthropology* 33:179–97.
Advantage Business Media
   2006 "Phase 3 Clinical Trial Costs Exceed $26,000 Per Patient." *Pharmaceutical
      Processing*, 1 November. *highbeam.com/doc/1G1-155782894.html.*
Allen, Caroline F., Nicola Desmond, Betty Chiduo, Lemmy Medard, Shelley S. Lees,
Andrew Vallely, Suzanna C. Francis, David A. Ross, and Richard J. Hayes
   2010 "Intravaginal and Menstrual Practices among Women Working in
      Food and Recreational Facilities in Mwanza, Tanzania: Implications for
      Microbicide Trials." *AIDS and Behavior* 14(5): 1169–81.
Allen, Tim
   2006 "AIDS and Evidence: Interrogating Some Ugandan Myths." *Journal of
      Biosocial Sciences* 38:7–28.
Allen, Tim, and Suzette Heald
   2004 "HIV/AIDS Policy in Africa: What Has Worked in Uganda and What
      Has Failed in Botswana?" *Journal of International Development* 16:1141–54.
Amadiume, Ifi
   2006 "Sexuality, African Religio-Cultural Traditions and Modernity: Expanding
      the Lens." *CODESRIA Bulletin* 1 & 2: 26–28.
Arikha, Noga
   2007 *Passions and Tempers: A History of the Humours.* New York: Ecco.

Ashforth, Adam
    2005   *Witchcraft, Violence, and Democracy in South Africa*. Chicago: University of
        Chicago Press.
Auerbach, Judith
    2013   "CROI 2013: The VOICE Results—A Social Scientist's Perspective."
        Interview by Reilly O'Neal. *BETA*, 13 March. *betablog.org*.
Bagnol, Brigitte, and Esmeralda Mariano
    2008   "Vaginal Practices: Eroticism and Implications for Women's Health and
        Condom Use in Mozambique." *Culture, Health & Sexuality* 10(6): 573–85.
Bähre, Erik
    2002   "Witchcraft and the Exchange of Sex, Blood, and Money among Africans
        in Cape Town, South Africa." *Journal of Religion in Africa* 32(3): 300–335.
Bass, Emily
    2002   "Learning from Microbicides: A Young Field's Experience Working with
        High-Risk Women." *AIDScience* 2(17).
BBC News
    2002   "Seaweed Gel Could Protect against HIV." *BBC News*, 2 February. *news.
        bbc.co.uk*.
    2008   "No Clinical Trials for SA Healers." *BBC News*, 24 February. *news.bbc.
        co.uk*.
Beecher, Henry K.
    1966   "Ethics and Clinical Research." *New England Journal of Medicine*
        274:1354–60.
Beksinska, Mags E., Helen V. Rees, Immo Kleinschmidt, and James McIntyre
    1999   "The Practice and Prevalence of Dry Sex among Men and Women in
        South Africa: A Risk Factor for Sexually Transmitted Infections?" *Sexually
        Transmitted Infections* 75:178–80.
Bell, Susan E.
    2000   "Accéder au pouvoir par les technologies: Femmes et science dans la
        recherche sur les microbicides" (Empowering technologies: Connecting
        women and science in microbicide research). *Sciences Sociales et Sante*
        18:121–40.
    2003   "Sexual Synthetics: Women, Science and Microbicides." In *Synthetic
        Planet: Chemical Politics and the Hazards of Modern Life*. M. J. Casper, ed.
        Pp. 197–211. London: Routledge.
Bentley, Margaret E., Andrew M. Fullem, Elizabeth E. Tolley,
Clifton W. Kelly, Neelam Jogelkar, Namtip Srirak, Liness Mwafulirwa,
Gertrude Khumalo-Sakutukwa, and David D. Celentano
    2004   "Acceptability of a Microbicide among Women and Their Partners in a
        4-Country Phase I Trial." *American Journal of Public Health* 94:1159–64.

Bermudes Ribiero Da Cruz, Claudia C.

2004 "From Policy to Practice: The Anthropology of Condom Use." In *AIDS and South Africa: The Social Expression of a Pandemic*. Kyle D. Kauffman and David L. Lindauer, eds. Pp. 136–60. Hampshire, UK: Palgrave Macmillan.

Besnier, Nico

1994 "The Truth and Other Irrelevant Aspects of Nukulaelae Gossip." *Pacific Studies* 17(3): 1–39.

Bhatt, Arun

2010 "Pragmatic Fact-Making: Contracts and Contexts in the UK and the Gambia." *Perspectives in Clinical Research* 1(1): 6–10.

Bibeau, Gilles, and Duncan Pedersen

2002 "A Return to Scientific Racism in Medical Social Sciences: The Case of Sexuality and the AIDS Epidemic in Africa." In *New Horizons in Medical Anthropology: Essays in Honor of Charles Leslie*. M. Nichter and M. Lock, eds. Pp. 141–71. New York: Routledge.

Biehl, João

2009 *Will to Live: AIDS Therapies and the Politics of Survival*. Princeton, NJ: Princeton University Press.

Bland, Ruth M., Nigel C. Rollins, Jan Van den Broeck,
Hoosen M. Coovadia, and Child Health Group

2004 "The Use of Non-Prescribed Medication in the First 3 Months of Life in Rural South Africa." *Tropical Medicine & International Health* 9(1): 118–24.

Boahene, Kwasi

1996 "The IXth International Conference on AIDS and STDs in Africa." *AIDS Care* 8(5): 609–16.

Boas, Franz

1904 "Some Traits of Primitive Culture." *Journal of American Folklore* 17(67): 243–54.

1911 *The Mind of Primitive Man*. New York: Macmillan.

Bonner, Philip, and Lauren Segal

1998 *Soweto: A History*. Cape Town: Maskew, Miller and Longman.

Boonstra, Heather D.

2000 "Campaign to Accelerate Microbicide Development for STD Prevention Gets Under Way." *Guttmacher Report on Public Policy* 3(1).

Boseley, Sarah

2009 "Anti-HIV Gel Hopes Dashed by Trial Results: Promising Microbicide Piloted in British-Funded Trial Turns Out to Be Ineffective." *Guardian*, 14 December. *theguardian.com*.

Braun, Virginia, and Celia Kitzinger

2001 "The Perfectible Vagina: Size Matters." *Culture, Health & Sexuality* 3(3): 263–77.

Briggs, Charles L.
  2005 "Communicability, Racial Discourse, and Disease." *Annual Review of Anthropology* 34:269–91.
Briggs, Charles, and Clara Mantini-Briggs
  2004 *Stories in the Time of Cholera*. Berkeley: University of California Press.
Brown, Judith E., Okako Bibi Ayowa, and Richard C. Brown
  1993 "Dry and Tight: Sexual Practices and Potential AIDS Risk in Zaire." *Social Science & Medicine* 37(8): 989–94.
Brown, Judith E., and Richard C. Brown
  2000 "Traditional Intravaginal Practices and the Heterosexual Transmission of Disease: A Review." *Sexually Transmitted Diseases* 27(4): 183–87.
Burke, Timothy
  1996 *Lifebuoy Men, Lux Women: Commodification, Consumption, and Cleanliness in Modern Zimbabwe*. Berkeley: University of California Press.
Caldwell, John C., Pat Caldwell, and Pat Quiggin
  1989 "The Social Context of AIDS in Sub-Saharan Africa." *Population and Development Review* 15(2): 185–234.
Campbell, T., and M. Kelly
  1995 "Women and AIDS in Zambia: A Review of the Psychosocial Factors Implicated in the Transmission of HIV." *AIDS Care* 7(3): 365–73.
Cassell, Joan
  2002 "Perturbing the System: 'Hard Science,' 'Soft Science,' and Social Science, The Anxiety and Madness of Method." *Human Organization* 61(2): 177–85.
Campion-Vincent, Véronique
  2002 "Organ Theft Narratives as Medical and Social Critique." *Journal of Folklore Research* 39(1): 33–50.
Chalmers, Iain, and Mike Clarke
  2004 "The 1944 Patulin Trial: The First Properly Controlled Multicentre Trial Conducted under the Aegis of the British Medical Research Council." *International Journal of Epidemiology* 32:253–60.
Check, Erika
  2007 "HIV Trial Doomed by Design, Say Critics." *Nature* 448(7150): 110–11.
Chersich, Matthew F., and Helen Rees
  2008 "Vulnerability of Women in Southern Africa to Infection with HIV: Biological Determinants and Priority Health Sector Interventions." *AIDS* 22(Supplement 4): S1–S14.
Chimbiri, Agnes M.
  2007 "The Condom Is an 'Intruder' in Marriage: Evidence from Rural Malawi." *Social Science & Medicine* 64:1102–15.

Chipfakacha, V. G.

1997 "STD/HIV/AIDS Knowledge, Beliefs and Practices of Traditional Healers in Botswana." *AIDS Care* 9(4): 417–25.

Citizen News Service

2009 "Microbicide Trial Results Signal End of One Chapter, Focus Turns to Promising ARV-Based Candidates." *Citizen News Service*, 24 December. *citizen-news.org*.

Civic, Diane, and David Wilson

1996 "Dry Sex in Zimbabwe and Implications for Condom Use." *Social Science & Medicine* 42(1): 91–98.

Cleland, John G., and Benoît Ferry

1995 *Sexual Behavior and AIDS in the Developing World*. London: Taylor & Francis.

Cohen, Jon

2013 "Human Nature Sinks HIV Prevention Trial." *Science*, 7 March. *news. sciencemag.org*.

Collins, Terri, and Jonathan Stadler

2000 "Love, Passion and Play: Sexual Meaning among Youth in the Northern Province of South Africa." *Journal des Anthropologues* 82:325–38.

Comaroff, Jean

1985 *Body of Power, Spirit of Resistance: The Culture and History of a South African People*. Chicago: University of Chicago Press.

1993 "The Diseased Heart of Africa: Medicine, Colonialism, and the Black Body." In *Knowledge, Power, and Practice: The Anthropology of Medicine and Everyday Life*. S. Lindenbaum and M. Lock, eds. Pp. 305–29. Berkeley: University of California Press.

Comaroff, Jean, and John Comaroff

1991 *Of Revelation and Revolution*. Vol. 1, *Christianity, Colonialism, and Consciousness in South Africa*. Chicago: University of Chicago Press.

1992 *Ethnography and the Historical Imagination*. Boulder, CO: Westview Press.

1997 *Of Revelation and Revolution*. Vol. 2, *The Dialectics of Modernity on a South African Frontier*. Chicago: University of Chicago Press.

1999 "Occult Economies and the Violence of Abstraction: Notes from the South African Postcolony." *American Ethnologist* 26(2): 279–303.

2000 "Millenial Capitalism: First Thoughts on the Second Coming." *Public Culture* 12(2): 1–35.

2011 *Theory from the South: Or, How Euro-America Is Evolving toward Africa*. New York: Paradigm.

Cornwall, Andrea

   2002  "Spending Power: Love, Money, and the Reconfiguration of Gender
      Relations in Ado-Odo, Southwestern Nigeria." *American Ethnologist* 29(4):
      963–80.

Craddock, Susan

   2004  "AIDS and Ethics: Clinical Trials, Pharmaceuticals, and Global Scientific
      Practice." In *HIV and AIDS in Africa: Beyond Epidemiology*. E. Kalipeni, S.
      Craddock, J. Oppong, and J. Ghosh, eds. Pp. 240–51. Oxford: Blackwell.

Crandon-Malamud, Libbet

   1993  *From the Fat of Our Souls: Social Change, Political Process, and Medical
      Pluralism in Bolivia*. Berkeley: University of California Press.

Crankshaw, Owen

   1993  "Squatting, Apartheid and Urbanisation on the Southern Witwatersrand."
      *African Affairs* 92(366): 31–51.

   2005  "Class, Race and Residence in Black Johannesburg, 1923–1970." *Journal
      of Historical Sociology* 18(4): 353–93.

Crankshaw, Owen, Alan Gilbert, and Alan Morris

   2000  "Backyard Soweto." *International Journal of Urban and Regional Research*
      24(4): 841–57.

Crankshaw, Owen, and Timothy Hart

   1990  *The Human and Social Impacts of the Squatter Relocation to Orange Farm*.
      Pretoria: Human Sciences Research Council.

Crapanzano, Vincent

   2003  "Reflections on Hope as a Category of Social and Psychological Analysis."
      *Cultural Anthropology* 18(1): 3–32.

Crofton, J.

   2006  "The MRC Randomized Trial of Streptomycin and its Legacy: A View
      from the Clinical Front Line." *Journal of the Royal Society of Medicine* 99(10):
      531–34.

Curry, Jen

   2003  "The International Epidemiologist: A Talk with Zena Stein." *Gay Men's
      Health Crisis*, September. *thebody.com/content/art13228.html*.

Daily Mail

   2010  "The Condom with TEETH: South African Doctor Designs New Female
      Contraceptive to Ward Off Would-Be Rapists." *Daily Mail* (London), 21
      June. *dailymail.co.uk/news/article-1288133*.

De Heusch, Luc

   1980  "Heat, Physiology, and Cosmogony: Rites of Passage among the Thonga."
      In *Explorations in African Systems of Thought*. I. Karp and C. S. Bird, eds.
      Pp. 28–43. Bloomington: University of Indiana Press.

Dehue, Trudy
    2010 "Pragmatic Fact-Making: Contracts and Contexts in the UK and the
        Gambia." In *Medical Proofs, Social Experiments: Clinical Trials in Shifting
        Contexts*. C. Will and T. Moreira, eds. Pp. 103–21. London: Ashgate.
Delany-Moretlwe, Sinead, Ananta Nanoo,
Ameet S. Nagpal, Harry Moultrie, and Helen Rees
    2011 "P1-S5.14 Risk Factors Associated with HIV Acquisition: A Comparative
        Analysis of Older and Younger Women Who Participated in the MDP301
        Trial in Johannesburg." *Sexually Transmitted Infections* 87(Supplement 1):
        A179–A180.
Delany-Moretlwe, Sinead, Jonathan Stadler, Philippe Mayaud, and Helen Rees
    2011 "Investing in the Future: Lessons Learnt from Communicating the Results
        of HSV/ HIV Intervention Trials in South Africa." *Health Research Policy and
        Systems* 9(Supplement 1).
DelVecchio Good, Mary-Jo
    2001 "The Biotechnical Embrace." *Culture, Medicine and Psychiatry* 25(4):
        395–410.
    2007 "The Medical Imaginary and the Biotechnical Embrace: Subjective
        Experiences of Clinical Scientists and Patients." In *Subjectivity: Ethnographic
        Investigations*. J. Biehl, B. Good, and A. Kleinman, eds. Pp. 362–80.
        Berkeley: University of California Press.
Department of Health
    1997 "Towards a National Health System." White paper for the Transformation
        of the Health System in South Africa. Pretoria: Department of Health.
De Wet, Thea, Leila Patel, Marcel Korth, and Chris Forrester
    2008 *Johannesburg Poverty and Livelihoods Study*. Johannesburg: Centre for
        Social Development in Africa, University of Johannesburg.
Douglas, Mary
    1966 *Purity and Danger: An Analysis of Concepts of Pollution and Taboo*. New York:
        Routledge.
Dumit, Joseph
    2012 *Drugs for Life: How Pharmaceutical Companies Define Our Health*.
        Durham, NC: Duke University Press.
Dunkle, Kristin L., Rachel K. Jewkes, Heather C. Brown,
Glenda E. Gray, James A. McIntyre, and Siobán D. Harlow
    2004a "Gender-Based Violence, Relationship Power, and Risk of HIV Infection
        in Women Attending Antenatal Clinics in South Africa." *Lancet* 363 (9419):
        1415–21.
    2004b "Transactional Sex among Women in Soweto, South Africa: Prevalence,
        Risk Factors and Association with HIV Infection." *Social Science & Medicine*
        59:1581–92.

Dunn, J. P., J. E. Krige, R. Wood, P. C. Bornman, and J. Terreblanche
    1991 "Colonic Complications after Toxic Tribal Enemas." *British Journal of Surgery* 78(5): 545–48.
Elias, Christopher J., and Lori Heise
    1993 "The Development of Microbicides: A New Method of HIV Prevention for Women." Working paper 6. New York: Population Council.
Epstein, Steven
    1995 "The Construction of Lay Expertise: AIDS Activism and the Forging of Credibility in the Reform of Clinical Trials." *Science, Technology, & Human Values* 20(4): 408–37.
    1997 "Activism, Drug Regulation, and the Politics of Therapeutic Evaluation in the AIDS Era: A Case Study of DDC and the 'Surrogate Markers' Debate." *Social Studies of Science* 27:691–726.
Etkin, Nina L.
    1988 "Cultural Constructions of Efficacy." In *The Context of Medicines in Developing Countries*. S. van der Geest and S. R. Whyte, eds. Pp. 299–326. Boston: Kluwer Academic Publishers.
    1992 "'Side Effects': Cultural Constructions and Reinterpretations of Western Pharmaceuticals." *Medical Anthropology Quarterly* 6(2): 99–113.
Evans-Pritchard, E. E.
    1974 *Man and Woman among the Azande*. New York: Free Press.
Fairhead, James, Melissa Leach, and Mary Small
    2006 "Public Engagement with Science? Local Understandings of a Vaccine Trial in the Gambia." *Journal of Biosocial Science* 38(1): 103–16.
Farley, John
    1991 *Bilharzia: A History of Imperial Tropical Medicine*. Cambridge: Cambridge University Press.
Fassin, Didier
    2006 "The End of Ethnography as Collateral Damage of Ethical Regulation?" *American Ethnologist* 33:522–24.
    2007 *When Bodies Remember: Experiences and Politics of AIDS in South Africa*. Berkeley: University of California Press.
Ferguson, James
    1990 *The Anti-Politics Machine: "Development," Depoliticization and Bureaucratic State Power in Lesotho*. Cambridge: Cambridge University Press.
FHI (Family Health International)
    2008 *Technical Report: Behavioral and Social Science Support to CONRAD Phase III Clinical Trial of Cellulose Sulfate 6% Gel*. Research Triangle Park, NC: FHI.

FHI 360

    2012 "FHI 360 Senior Scientist Lut Van Damme Receives International Microbicide Conference Lifetime Achievement Award." *FHI 360 News*, April 19.

Fisher, Jill

    2008 *Medical Research for Hire: The Political Economy of Pharmaceutical Clinical Trials*. New Brunswick, NJ: Rutgers University Press.

Fleming, Mike

    2000 "Ban Called for on Nonoxynol-9 Products: Spermicide May Promote HIV Infection, Leading Experts to Urge Discontinuation of Use by Gay Men." *Washington Blade*, 4 October. *www.global-campaign.org/clientfiles/Blade.pdf*.

Flint, Austin

    1863 "A Contribution toward the Natural History of Articular Rheumatism, Consisting of a Report of Thirteen Cases Treated Solely with Palliative Measures." *American Journal of Medical Sciences* 46(July): 17–36.

Forbes, Anna

    2010 "Leaving the Global Campaign: Anna Forbes' Parting Thoughts." *GC News* 118 (4 February): 1–2.

Foss, Anna M., Peter T. Vickerman, Lori Heise, and Charlotte H. Watts

    2003 "Shifts in Condom Use Following Microbicide Introduction: Should We Be Concerned?" *AIDS* 17(8):1227–37.

Foucault, Michel

    1994 *The Birth of the Clinic: An Archaeology of Medical Perception*. New York: Vintage.

Fox, Renee C., and Judith P. Swazey

    1984 "Medical Morality Is Not Bioethics—Medical Ethics in China and the United States." *Perspectives in Biology and Medicine* 27:336–60.

Gafos, Mitzy, Misiwe Mzimela, Hlengiwe Ndlovu, Nkosinathi Mhlongo, Yael Hoogland, and Richard Mutemwa

    2011 "'One Teabag Is Better Than Four': Participants Response to the Discontinuation of 2 percent PRO 2000/5 Microbicide Gel in KwaZulu-Natal, South Africa." *PLoS ONE* 6(1).

Gafos, Mitzy, Misiwe Mzimela, Sizakele Sukazi, Robert Pool, Catherine Montgomery, and Jonathan Elford

    2010 "Intravaginal Insertion in KwaZulu-Natal: Sexual Practices and Preferences in the Context of Microbicide Gel Use." *Culture, Health & Sexuality* 12(8): 929–42.

Gausset, Quentin

    2001 "AIDS and Cultural Practices in Africa: The Case of the Tonga (Zambia)." *Social Science & Medicine* 52:509–18.

GCM (Global Campaign for Microbicides)

2002   "Campaign Honors Its First Mrs. McCormick." *Global Campaign for Microbicides and Prevention Options for Women Update* 1(2): 2.

2006   "Why Women Should NOT Use Lemon or Lime Juice as a Microbicide" (information sheet). June. *global-campaign.org/clientfiles/New-Lemon-Lime_June24.pdf.*

2011   "Advocacy in Action." *Global Campaign News*, July. *global-campaign.org.*

2016   "About Microbicides." Global Campaign for Microbicides, accessed 3 May. *global-campaign.org.*

Geary, Cynthia W., and Elizabeth A. Bukusi

2014   "Women and ARV-Based Prevention: Opportunities and Challenges." *Journal of the International AIDS Society* 17(3 Supplement 2).

Geissler, Paul Wenzel

2005a   "Kachinja Are Coming!: Encounters around Medical Research Work in a Kenyan Village." *Africa* 75(2): 173–202.

2005b   "Blood-Stealing Rumours in Western Kenya: A Local Critique of Medical Research in Its Global Context." In *Managing Uncertainty: Ethnographic Studies of Illness, Risk, and the Struggle for Control.* R. Jenkins, H. Jessen, and V. Steffen, eds. Pp. 123–48. Copenhagen: Museum Tusculanum Press.

Geissler, Paul Wenzel, Ann Kelly, Babatunde Imoukhuede, and Robert Pool

2008   "'He Is Now Like a Brother, I Can Even Give Him Some Blood'— Relational Ethics and Material Exchanges in a Malaria Vaccine 'Trial Community' in the Gambia." *Social Science & Medicine* 67(5): 696–707.

Gilbert, Alan, and Owen Crankshaw

1999   "Comparing South African and Latin American Experience: Migration and Housing Mobility in Soweto." *Urban Studies* 36:2375–2400.

Gilman, Sander L.

1985   "Black Bodies, White Bodies: Toward an Iconography of Female Sexuality in Late Nineteenth-Century Art, Medicine, and Literature." *Critical Inquiry* 12(1): 204–42.

Glaser, Clive

2000   *Bo-Tsotsi. The Youth Gangs of Soweto, 1935–1976.* Oxford: James Currey.

Goeman, Johan, Ibra Ndoye, Lamine M. Sakho,

Souleymane Mboup, Peter Piot, Marc Karam, Elizabeth Belsey,

Joep M. A. Lange, Marie Laga, and Joseph H. Perriëns

1995   "Frequent Use of Menfegol Spermicidal Vaginal Foaming Tablets Associated with a High Incidence of Genital Lesions." *Journal of Infectious Diseases* 171(6): 1611–14.

Gordon, Deborah

1988 "Tenacious Assumptions in Western Medicine." In *Biomedicine Examined*. M. Lock and D. Gordon, eds. Pp. 19–56. Dordrecht, Netherlands: Kluwer Academic Publishers.

Grant, Robert M., Dean Hamer, Thomas Hope, Rowena Johnston, Joep Lange, Michael M. Lederman, Judy Lieberman, et al.

2008 "Whither or Wither Microbicides?" *Science* 321(5888): 532–34.

Graves, Joseph

2001 *The Emperor's New Clothes: Biological Theories of Race at the Millennium.* New Brunswick, NJ: Rutgers University Press.

Green, Edward C.

1999 *Indigenous Theories of Contagious Disease.* Walnut Creek, CA: AltaMira Press.

Grosz, Elizabeth

1994 *Volatile Bodies: Toward a Corporeal Feminism.* Bloomington: Indiana University Press.

Gupta, Geeta Rao, and Ellen Weiss

1993 "Women's Lives and Sex: Implications for AIDS Prevention." *Culture, Medicine and Psychiatry* 17(4): 399–412.

Haire, Bridget, John Kaldor, and Christopher F. C. Jordens

2012 "How Good Is 'Good Enough'? The Case for Varying Standards of Evidence According to Need for New Interventions in HIV Prevention." *American Journal of Bioethics* 12(6): 21–30.

Hammond-Tooke, William David

1981 *Boundaries and Belief: The Structure of a Sotho Worldview.* Johannesburg: Witwatersrand University Press.

1989 *Rituals and Medicines: Indigenous Healing in South Africa.* Johannesburg: A. D. Donker.

Hardon, Anita

2012 "The Turn to Female-Controlled Safe Sex Technologies." In *Technologies of Sexuality, Identity and Sexual Health*. L. Manderson, ed. Pp. 55–72. Oxon, UK: Routledge.

Harkness, Jon

1996 "Nuremberg and the Issue of Wartime Experiments on US Prisoners: The Green Committee." *Journal of the American Medical Association* 276:1672–75.

Harkness, Jon, Susan E. Lederer, and Daniel Wikler

2001 "Laying the Ethical Foundation for Clinical Research." *Bulletin of the World Health Organization* 79(4): 365–66.

Harries, A. D., D. S. Nyangulu, N. J. Hargreaves, O. Kaluwa, and F. M. Salaniponi
   2001  "Preventing Antiretroviral Anarchy in sub-Saharan Africa." *Lancet*
      358(9279): 410–14.

Harrison, Polly F.
   1999  "A New Model for Collaboration: The Alliance for Microbicide
      Development." *International Journal of Gynaecology and Obstetrics*
      67:S39–S53.
   2011  "The Past, Present, and Future of HIV Microbicide Research Advocacy:
      An Interview with Polly Harrison, Founder of the Alliance for Microbicide
      Development," by Treatment Action Group. *TAGline* 18:1–4.

Hearst, Norman, and Sanny Chen
   2004  "Condom Promotion for AIDS Prevention in the Developing World: Is It
      Working?" *Studies in Family Planning* 35(1): 39–47.

Heise, Lori
   2009  *Microbicides: The Herstory of a Movement.* Teleconference presentation,
      International Rectal Microbicide Advocates, 11 June.
   2016  Interview. AVAC: Global Advocacy for HIV Prevention. Accessed 13 July.
      *avac.org/lori-heise-interview.*

Heise, Lori L., Charlotte Watts, Anna Foss, James Trussell,
Peter Vickerman, Richard Hayes, and Sheena McCormack
   2011  "Apples and Oranges? Interpreting Success in HIV Prevention Trials."
      *Contraception* 83(1): 10–15.

Hemmings, Colin P.
   2005  "Rethinking Medical Anthropology: How Anthropology Is Failing
      Medicine." *Anthropology & Medicine* 12(2): 91–103.

Henderson, Patricia C.
   2004  "The Vertiginous Body and the Social Metamorphosis in a Context of
      HIV/AIDS." *Anthropology Southern Africa* 27(1&2): 43–53.

Herman, Robin
   1998  "In the Developing World the Female Condom Is No Joke." *Washington
      Post*, 8 July.

Hilber, Adriane Martin, Elise Kenter, Shelagh Redmond,
Sonja Merten, Brigitte Bagnol, Nicola Lowa, and Ruth Garside
   2012  "Vaginal Practices as Women's Agency in Sub-Saharan Africa: A Synthesis
      of Meaning and Motivation through Meta-Ethnography." *Social Science &
      Medicine* 74:1311–23.

HIV Vaccines and Microbicides Resource Tracking Working Group
   2008  *Sustaining the HIV Prevention Research Agenda: Funding for Research and
      Development of HIV Vaccines, Microbicides and Other New Prevention Options,
      2000 to 2007.* New York: AVAC. *hivresourcetracking.org.*

2013 *From Research to Reality: Investing in HIV Prevention Research in a Challenging Landscape.* New York: AVAC.

Hlongwa, Wonder

2007a "Concern over HIV Trial Researcher's Workload." *Johannesburg City Press*, 11 February. *152.111.1.87/argief/berigte/citypress/2007/02/11/CP/1/whaidstrials.html.*

2007b "Medical Research Trial Guinea Pigs Contract HIV." *Johannesburg City Press*, 4 February. *152.111.1.87/argief/berigte/citypress/2007/02/04/CP/1/mkmicro.html.*

Hoad, Neville

2005 "Thabo Mbeki's AIDS Blues: The Intellectual, the Archive and the Pandemic." *Public Culture* 17:101–27.

Hull, Terence, Adriane Martin Hilber, Matthew F. Chersich, Brigitte Bagnol, Aree Prohmmo, Jennifer A. Smit, Ninuk Widyantoro, Iwu Dwisetyani Utomo, Isabelle Franc, Nazarius Mbona Tumwesigye, and Marleen Temmerman

2011 "Prevalence, Motivations, and Adverse Effects of Vaginal Practices in Africa and Asia: Findings from a Multicountry Household Survey." *Journal of Women's Health* 20(7): 1097–1109.

Hunter, Mark

2002 "The Materiality of Everyday Sex: Thinking beyond 'Prostitution.'" *African Studies* 61(1): 99–120.

ICH (International Conference on Harmonisation of Technical Requirements for Registration of Pharmaceuticals for Human Use)

1996 *Guideline for Good Clinical Practice.* Geneva: ICH. *ich.org.*

Iliffe, John

2006 *The African AIDS Epidemic: A History.* Cape Town: Double Storey.

IRIN

2007 "Clarity Sought in Microbicides Furore." IRIN, 7 February. *irinnews.org.*

2010 "South Africa: Communities Debate Microbicide Results." IRIN, 23 August, *irinnews.org.*

Jellinek, Elvin Morton

1946 "Clinical Tests on Comparative Effectiveness of Analgesic Drugs." *Biometrics Bulletin* 2(5): 87–91.

Jewkes, Rachel, and Kate Wood

1999 "Problematizing Pollution: Dirty Wombs, Ritual Pollution and Pathological Processes." *Medical Anthropology* 18:163–86.

Jewkes, Rachel, Jonathan B. Levin, and Loveday Penn-Kekana

2002 "Risk Factors for Domestic Violence: Findings from a South African Cross-Sectional Study." *Social Science & Medicine* 55:1603–17.

2003 "Gender Inequalities, Intimate Partner Violence and HIV Preventive Practices: Findings of a South African Cross-Sectional Study." *Social Science & Medicine* 56:125–34.

Jochelson, Karen
2001 *The Colour of Disease: Syphilis and Racism in South Africa, 1880–1950.* New York: Palgrave.

Joint United Nations Programme on HIV/AIDS
2014 *The Gap Report 2014: People Living with HIV/AIDS.* Geneva: Joint United Nations Programme on HIV/AIDS.

Jones, James
1993 *Bad Blood: The Tuskegee Syphilis Experiment.* New and expanded edition. New York: Free Press.

Kaler, Amy
2004 "The Female Condom in North America: Selling the Technology of 'Empowerment.'" *Journal of Gender Studies* 13(2).
2006 "'When They See Money, They Think It's Life': Money, Modernity and Morality in Two Sites in Rural Malawi." *Journal of Southern African Studies* 32(2): 335–49.
2009 "Health Interventions and the Persistence of Rumour: The Circulation of Sterility Stories in African Public Health Campaigns." *Social Science & Medicine* 68(9): 1711–19.

Kalichman, Seth, Lisa Eaton, and Steven Pinkerton
2007 "Circumcision for HIV Prevention: Failure to Fully Account for Behavioral Risk Compensation." *PLoS Medicine* 4(3): e138.

Karim, Quarraisha Abdool, Hilton Humphries, and Zena Stein
2012 "Empowering Women in Human Immunodeficiency Virus Prevention." *Best Practice & Research Clinical Obstetrics & Gynaecology* 26:487–93.

Karim, Quarraisha Abdool, Salim S. Abdool Karim, Janet A. Frohlich, Anneke C. Grobler, Cheryl Baxter, Leila E. Mansoor, Ayesha B. M. Kharsany, Sengeziwe Sibeko, Koleka P. Mlisana, Zaheen Omar, Tanuja N. Gengiah, Silvia Maarschalk, Natasha Arulappan, Mukelisiwe Mlotshwa, Lynn Morris, and Douglas Taylor
2010 "Effectiveness and Safety of Tenofovir Gel, an Antiretroviral Microbicide, for the Prevention of HIV Infection in Women." *Science* 329:1168–74.

Karim, Salim S. Abdool, Barbra A. Richardson, Gita Ramjee, Irving F. Hoffman, Zvavahera M Chirenje, Taha Taha, Muzala Kapina, Lisa Maslankowski, Anne Coletti, Albert Profy, Thomas R. Moench, Estelle Piwowar-Manning, Benoît Mâsse, Sharon L. Hillier, and Lydia Soto-Torres, on behalf of the HPTN 035 Study Team
2011 "Safety and Effectiveness of BufferGel and 0.5% PRO 2000 Gel for the Prevention of HIV Infection in Women." *AIDS* 25(7): 957.

Karpas, Abraham
1987 "Origin of the AIDS Virus Explained?" *New Scientist*, July, 67.

Kaufman, Carol, and Stavros E. Stavrou

2002 "Bus Fare, Please: The Economics of Sex and Gifts among Adolescents in Urban South Africa." Policy Research Division working paper. New York: Population Council.

Klaits, Frederick

2010 *Death in a Church of Life: Moral Passion during Botswana's Time of AIDS.* Berkeley: University of California Press.

Kleinman, Arthur

1980 *Patients and Healers in the Context of Culture: An Exploration of the Borderland between Anthropology, Medicine, and Psychiatry.* Berkeley: University of California Press.

Kleinman, Arthur, and Peter Benson

2006 "Culture, Moral Experience, and Medicine." *Mount Sinai Journal of Medicine* 73(6): 834–41.

Krige, Detlev

2011 "Power, Identity and Agency at Work in the Popular Economies of Soweto and Black Johannesburg," PhD thesis, University of the Witwatersrand.

Kristeva, Julia

1982 *Powers of Horror: An Essay in Abjection.* L. Roudiez, transl. New York: Columbia University Press.

Kun, Karen E.

1998 "Vaginal Drying Agents and HIV Transmission." *International Family Planning Perspectives* 24(2): 93–94.

Kuper, Adam

1999 *Culture: The Anthropologists' Account.* Cambridge, MA: Harvard University Press.

Kutikuppala, S. R., R. Rajeswari, and P. Ramadevi

2004 "Microbicides and Empowerment of Women in Developing Countries in HIV and STI Prevention." Abstract no. TuPeB4660. 15th International Conference on AIDS, Bangkok, 11–16 July.

Leclerc-Madlala, Suzanne

2001a "Demonising Women in the Era of AIDS: On the Relationship between Cultural Constructions of both HIV/AIDS and Femininity." *Society in Transition* 32(1): 38–46.

2001b "Virginity Testing: Managing Sexuality in a Maturing HIV/AIDS Epidemic." *Medical Anthropology Quarterly* 15(4): 533–52.

2002 "On the Virgin Cleansing Myth: Gendered Bodies, AIDS and Ethnomedicine." *African Journal of AIDS Research* 1:87–95.

2003 "Transactional Sex and the Pursuit of Modernity." *Social Dynamics* 29(2): 213–33.

Lederman, Michael M., Robin E. Offord, and Oliver Hartley
2006 "Microbicides and Other Topical Strategies to Prevent Vaginal Transmission of HIV." *Nature Reviews Immunology* 6(5): 371–82.

Lees, Shelley, Nicola Desmond, Caroline Allen,
Gilbert Bugeke, Andrew Vallely, and David Ross
2009 "Sexual Risk Behaviour for Women Working in Recreational Venues in Mwanza, Tanzania: Considerations for the Acceptability and Use of Vaginal Microbicide Gels." *Culture, Health & Sexuality* 11(6): 581–95.

Leger, Claire Marie
2008 "Clinical Globalization: A Case Study of Privately-Sponsored HIV Research in Mexico." *Social Identities* 14(2): 189–213.

LeMoncheck, Linda
1997 *Loose Women, Lecherous Men: A Feminist Philosophy of Sex*. Oxford: Oxford University Press.

Levin, Roy J.
2005 "Wet and Dry Sex—the Impact of Cultural Influence in Modifying Vaginal Function." *Sexual and Relationship Therapy* 20(4): 465–74.

Lewis, Stephen
2004 Speech at Microbicides 2004. London, 30 March. *data.unaids.org/GCWA/gcwa_sp_lewis_microbicides_30mar04_en.pdf*.

Löwy, Ileana
2000 "Trustworthy Knowledge and Desperate Patients: Clinical Tests for New Drugs from Cancer to AIDS." In *Living and Working with the New Medical Technologies: Intersections of Inquiry*. M. Lock, A. Young, and A. Cambrosio, eds. Pp. 49–81. Cambridge: Cambridge University Press.

Lusu, T., N. Buhlungu, and H. Grant
2001 "The Attitudes of Parents to Traditional Medicine and the Surgeon." *South African Medical Journal* 91(4): 270–71.

Lyons, Andrew E., and Harriet D. Lyons
2004 *Irregular Connections: A History of Anthropology and Sexuality*. Lincoln: University of Nebraska Press.

MacGregor, Hayley
2006 "'The Grant Is What I Eat': The Politics of Social Security and Disability in the Post-Apartheid South African State." *Journal of Biosocial Sciences* 38:43–55.

Mack, Natasha, Elizabeth T. Robinson, Kathleen M.
MacQueen, Jill Moffett, and Laura M. Johnson
2010 "The Exploitation of 'Exploitation' in the Tenofovir PrEP Trial in Cameroon: Lessons Learned from Media Coverage of an HIV Prevention Trial." *Journal of Empirical Research on Human Research Ethics* 5(2): 3–19.

Macleod, Catriona, and Kevin Durrheim
2002 "Racializing Teenage Pregnancy: 'Culture' and 'Tradition' in the South African Scientific Literature." *Ethnic and Racial Studies* 25(5): 778–801.

MacPhail, Catherine, and Catherine Campbell
2001 "'I Think Condoms Are Good but, Aai, I Hate Those Things': Condom Use Among Adolescents and Young People in a South African Township." *Social Science & Medicine* 52:1613–27.

Makiwane, Monde, Chris Desmond, Linda Richter, and Eric Udjo
2006 *Is the Child Support Grant Associated with an Increase in Teenage Fertility in South Africa? Evidence From National Surveys and Administrative Data.* Pretoria: Human Sciences Research Council.

Malik, Kenan
1996 *The Meaning of Race: Race, History, and Culture in Western Society.* Houndmills, UK: Macmillan.

Malow, R. M., D. Ziskind, and D. L. Jones
2000 "Use of Female Controlled Microbicidal Products for HIV Risk Reduction." *AIDS Care* 12:581–88.

Maman, Suzanne, Jacquelyn Campbell, Michael D. Sweat, and Andrea C. Gielen
2000 "The Intersection of HIV and Violence: Directions for Future Research and Interventions." *Social Science & Medicine* 50:459–78.

Manganyi, N. C.
1974 "Health and Disease: Some Topical Problems of Sociocultural Transition." *South African Medical Journal* 48(21): 922–24.

Mann, Jonathan, Nzila Nzilambi, Peter Piot, N. Bosenge, M. Kalala, Henry
Francis, R. C. Colebunders, P. K. Azila, James W. Curran, and Thomas C. Quinn
1988 "HIV Infection and Associated Risk Factors in Female Prostitutes in Kinshasa, Zaire." *AIDS* 2:249–54.

Mansoor, Leila Essop, Quarraisha Abdool Karim,
Nonhlanhla Yende-Zuma, Kathleen MacQueen, Cheryl Baxter,
Bernadette Madlala, Anneke Grobler, and Salim Abdool Karim
2014 "Adherence in the CAPRISA 004 Tenofovir Gel Microbicide Trial." *AIDS and Behavior* 4:1–9.

Mantell, Joanne E., Shari L. Dworkin, Theresa M. Exner,
Susie Hoffman, Jenni A. Smit, and Ida Susser
2006 "The Promises and Limitations of Female-Initiated Methods of HIV/STI Protection." *Social Science & Medicine* 63:1998–2009.

Mantell, Joanne E., Neetha S. Morar, Landon Myer, and Gita Ramjee
2006 "'We Have Our Protector': Misperceptions of Protection against HIV among Participants in a Microbicide Efficacy Trial." *American Journal of Public Health* 96(6): 1073–77.

Mantell, Joanne E., Landon Myer, Alex Carballo-Dieguez,
Zena Stein, Gita Ramjee, Neetha S. Morar, and Polly F. Harrison
    2005  "Microbicide Acceptability Research: Current Approaches and Future
        Directions." *Social Science & Medicine* 60:319–30.
Marks, Harry M.
    2000  *The Progress of Experiment: Science and Therapeutic Reform in the United
        States, 1900–1990.* Cambridge: Cambridge University Press.
Marrazzo, Jeane M., Gita Ramjee, Barbara A. Richardson, Kailazarid
Gomez, Nyaradzo Mgodi, Gonsagarie Nair, Thesla Palanee, Clemensia
Nakabiito, Ariane van der Straten, Lisa Noguchi, Craig W. Hendrix,
James Y. Dai, Shayhana Ganesh, Baningi Mkhize, Marthinette Taljaard,
Urvi M. Parikh, Jeanna Piper, Benoît Mâsse, Cynthia Grossman, James
Rooney, Jill L. Schwartz, Heather Watts, Mark A. Marzinke, Sharon L.
Hillier, Ian M. McGowan, Z. Mike Chirenje, and VOICE Study Team
    2015  "Tenofovir-Based Preexposure Prophylaxis for HIV Infection among
        African Women." *New England Journal of Medicine* 372(6): 509–18.
Mayer, Kenneth H., Salim Abdool Karim, Clifton Kelly, Lisa Maslankowski,
Helen Rees, Albert T. Profy, Jennifer Day, Julie Welch, and Zeda Rosenberg
    2003  "Safety and Tolerability of Vaginal PRO 2000 Gel in Sexually Active
        HIV-Uninfected and Abstinent HIV-Infected Women." *AIDS* 17(3):
        321–29.
Mbikusita-Lewanika, Mbololwa, Hart Stephen, and Jane Thomas
    2009  "The Prevalence of the Use of 'Dry Sex' Traditional Medicines, among
        Zambian Women, and the Profile of the Users." *Psychology, Health &
        Medicine* 14(2): 227–38.
McCormack, Sheena, Gita Ramjee, Anatoli Kamali,
Helen Rees, and Angela M. Crook
    2010  "PRO 2000 Vaginal Gel for Prevention of HIV-1 Infection (Microbicides
        Development Programme 301): A Phase 3, Randomised, Double-Blind,
        Parallel-Group Trial." *Lancet* 376(9749): 1329–37.
McGregor, Skye, Gilda Tachedjian, Bridget G. Haire, and John M. Kaldor
    2013  "The Seventh (and Last?) International Microbicides Conference: From
        Discovery to Delivery." *Sexual Health* 10(3): 240–45.
MDP (Microbicides Development Programme)
    2005  "More MDP Info." MDP. *www.mdp.mrc.ac.uk/more_info.html.*
    2008  "Q & A: Microbicides Development Programme (MDP) Update: MDP301
        Phase III Trial Continues But One Arm Closes" (PDF announcement). MDP,
        14 February. *www.mdp.mrc.ac.uk/archive.html.*
    2009a  "HIV 'Prevention' Gel PRO 2000 Proven Ineffective." MDP, 14
        December. *www.mdp.mrc.ac.uk/archive.html.*

2009b  "MDP 301 General Q&A" (PDF). MDP, 14 December. *www.mdp.mrc.ac.uk/archive.html.*

2009c  "MDP 301 Results Q&A" (PDF). MDP, 14 December. *www.mdp.mrc.ac.uk/archive.html.*

Medeossi, Bonnie-Jeanne, Jonathan Stadler, and Sinead Delany-Moretlwe
2014  "'I Heard about This Study on the Radio': Using Community Radio to Strengthen Good Participatory Practice in HIV Prevention Trials." *BMC Public Health* 14:876.

Mehendale, Sanjay, Swapna Deshpande, Rewa Kohli, Sharon Tsui, and Elizabeth Tolley
2012  "Acceptability of Coitally-Associated Versus Daily Use of 1% percent Tenofovir Vaginal Gel among Women in Pune, India." *International Health* 4(1): 63–69.

Mellors, John W., Barbara Richardson, Benoit R. Masse, Quarraisha A. Karim, Salim S. A. Karim, and Polly Harrison
2008  "Challenges in HIV-Prevention Microbicide Research." *Science* 321:532–34.

Middelthon, Anne-Lise
2001  "Interpretations of Condom Use and Nonuse among Young Norwegian Gay Men: A Qualitative Study." *Medical Anthropology Quarterly* 15(1): 58–83.

Mills, Elizabeth Anne
2006  "From the Physical Self to the Social Body: Expressions and Effects of HIV-Related Stigma in South Africa." *Journal of Community & Applied Social Psychology* 16(6): 498–503.

Minnis, Alexandra M., and Nancy S. Padian
2005  "Effectiveness of Female Controlled Barrier Methods in Preventing Sexually Transmitted Infections and HIV: Current Evidence and Future Research Directions." *Sexually Transmitted Infections* 81:193–200.

Minnis, Alexandra M., Markus J. Steiner, Maria F. Gallo, Lee Warner, Marcia M. Hobbs, Ariane Van der Straten, Tsungai Chipato, Maurizio Macaluso, and Nancy S. Padian
2009  "Biomarker Validation of Reports of Recent Sexual Activity: Results of a Randomized Controlled Study in Zimbabwe." *American Journal of Epidemiology* 170(7): 918–24.

Mngxitama, Andile
2010  "Research on HIV Prevention Gel Put Black Lives at Risk." *Sowetan Live*, 27 October. *sowetanlive.co.za.*

Moench, Thomas R., Deirdre E. O'Hanlon, and Richard A. Cone
2012  "Evaluation of Microbicide Gel Adherence Monitoring Methods." *Sexually Transmitted Diseases* 39(12).

Moffat, Robert
  1842 *Missionary Labours and Scenes in Southern Africa.* London: John Snow.
Moore, D. A., and N. L. Moore
  1998 "Paediatric Enema Syndrome in a Rural African Setting." *Annals of Tropical Paediatrics* 18(2): 139–44.
Morar, Neetha S., and Salim S. Abdool Karim
  1998 "Vaginal Insertion and Douching Practices among Sex Workers at Truck Stops in KwazuluNatal." *South African Medical Journal* 88(4): 470.
Morar, Neetha S., Gita Ramjee, Eleanor Gouws, and David Wilkinson
  2003 "Vaginal Douching and Vaginal Substance Use among Sex Workers in Kwazulu-Natal, South Africa." *South African Journal of Science* 99(July/August): 371–74.
Morris, Alan, and Belinda Bozzoli
  1999 *Change and Continuity: A Survey of Soweto in the Late 1990s.* Johannesburg: University of the Witwatersrand.
Morrow, Kathleen, Rochelle Rosen, Linda Richter, Anne Emans,
Anna Forbes, Jennifer Day, Neetha Morar, Lisa Maslankowski, Albert T.
Profy, Cliff Kelly, Salim S. Abdool Karim, and Kenneth H. Mayer
  2003 "The Acceptability of an Investigational Vaginal Microbicide, Pro 2000 Gel, among Women in a Phase I Clinical Trial." *Journal of Women's Health* 12(7): 655–66.
Murray, Colin
  1975 "Sex, Smoking and the Shades: A Sotho Symbolic Idiom." In *Religion and Social Change in Southern Africa: Anthropological Essays in Honour of Monica Wilson.* M. Whisson and M. West, eds. Pp. 58–77. Cape Town: David Philip.
  1981 *Families Divided: The Impact of Migrant Labour in Lesotho.* Cambridge: Cambridge University Press.
Myer, Landon, Lynette Denny, Michelle de Souza,
Thomas C. Wright, and Louise Kuhn
  2006 "Distinguishing the Temporal Association between Women's Intravaginal Practices and Risk of Human Immunodeficiency Virus Infection: A Prospective Study of South African Women." *American Journal of Epidemiology* 163(3): 552–60.
Myer, Landon, Louise Kuhn, Zena A. Stein,
Thomas C. Wright Jr., and Lynette Denny
  2005 "Intravaginal Practices, Bacterial Vaginosis, and Women's Susceptibility to HIV Infection: Epidemiological Evidence and Biological Mechanisms." *Lancet Infectious Disease* 5:786–94.

Nahmias, A. J., J. Weiss, X. Yao, F. Lee, R. Kodsi, M. Schanfield, T. Matthews,
D. Bolognesi, D. Durack, A. Motulsky, P. Kanki, and M. Essex
  1986 "Evidence for Human Infection with an HTLVIII/LAV-Like Virus in
    Central Africa, 1959." *Lancet* 327(8492): 1279.
Nattrass, Nicoli
  2007 *Mortal Combat: AIDS Denialism and the Struggle for Antiretrovirals in South
    Africa.* Durban: University of KwaZulu-Natal Press.
Newton, S., V. Doku, W. Geissler, K. Asante, and S. Cousens
  2009 "Drawing Blood from Young Children: Lessons Learned from a Trial in
    Ghana." *Transactions of the Royal Society of Tropical Medicine and Hygiene*
    103(5): 497–99.
Ngubane, Harriet
  1976 "Some Notions of 'Purity' and 'Impurity' among the Zulu." *Africa* 46(3):
    274–85.
  1977 *Body and Mind in Zulu Medicine: An Ethnography of Health and Disease in
    Nyuswa-Zulu Thought and Practice.* London: Academic Press.
Niehaus, Isak
  2000 "Coins for Blood and Blood for Coins: From Sacrifice to Ritual Murder in
    the South African Lowveld." *Etnofoor* 13(2): 31–54.
  2001 *Witchcraft, Power and Politics: Exploring the Occult in the South African
    Lowveld.* London: Pluto Press.
  2002 "Bodies, Heat and Taboos: Conceptualizing Modern Personhood in the
    South African Lowveld." *Ethnology* 41(3): 189–207.
Niehaus, Isak A., and Gunvor Jonsson
  2005 "Dr. Wouter Basson, Americans and Wild Beasts: Men's Conspiracy
    Theories of HIV/AIDS in the South African Lowveld." *Medical Anthropology*
    24:177–206.
Nundy, Samiran, and Chandra Gulhati
  2005 "A New Colonialism?—Conducting Clinical Trials in India." *New England
    Journal of Medicine* 352(16): 1633–36.
Nunn, Andrew, Sheena McCormack, Angela M. Crook,
Robert Pool, Clare Rutterford, and Richard Hayes
  2009 "Microbicides Development Programme: Design of a Phase III Trial
    to Measure the Efficacy of the Vaginal Microbicide PRO 2000/5 for HIV
    Prevention." *Trials* 10.
Nweneka, Chidi V.
  2007 *The Role of Advocacy in Advancing Microbicides Clinical Trials in Africa.*
    Presentation at the EDCTP (European and Developing Countries Clinical
    Trials Program) Stakeholders' Meeting on Microbicides, Oslo, Norway, 8 June.

Okal, Jerry, Jonathan Stadler, Wilkister Ombidi, Irene Jao,
Stanley Luchters, Marleen Temmerman, and Matthew F. Chersich
    2008 "Secrecy, Disclosure and Accidental Discovery: Perspectives of Diaphragm
        Users in Mombasa, Kenya." *Culture, Health & Sexuality* 10(1): 13–26.
Omar, Rabeea F., and Michel G. Bergeron
    2011 "The Future of Microbicides." *International Journal of Infectious Diseases*
        15(10): e656–e660.
Padian, Nancy S., Ariane van der Straten, Gita Ramjee, Tsungai Chipato,
Guy de Bruyn, Kelly Blanchard, Stephen Shiboski, Elizabeth T.
Montgomery, Heidi Fancher, Helen Cheng, Michael Rosenblum,
Mark van der Laan, Nicholas Jewell, James McIntyre, and Team MIRA
    2007 "Diaphragm and Lubricant Gel for Prevention of HIV Acquisition in
        Southern African Women: A Randomised Controlled Trial." *Lancet* 370(9583).
        *thelancet.com.*
Padian, Nancy S., Sandra I. McCoy, Jennifer E. Balkus, and Judith N. Wasserheit
    2010 "Weighing the Gold in the Gold Standard: Challenges in HIV Prevention
        Research." *AIDS* 24:621–35.
Patel, Leila, Tessa Hochfeld, Jacqueline Moodley, and Reem Mutwali
    2012 *The Gender Dynamics and Impact of the Child Support Grant in Doornkop,
        Soweto.* Johannesburg: Centre for Social Development in Africa, University of
        Johannesburg.
Pauw, B. A.
    1990 "Widows and Ritual Danger in Sotho and Tswana Communities." *African
        Studies* 49(2): 76–95.
Peltzer, Karl, Nolwandle Mngqundaniso, and George Petros
    2006 "HIV/AIDS/STI/TB Knowledge, Beliefs and Practices of Traditional
        Healers in KwaZulu-Natal, South Africa." *AIDS Care* 18(6): 608–13.
Peters, Anny J. T. P., Maja M. Scharf, Francien T. M.
van Driel, and Willy H. M. Jansen
    2010 "Where Does Public Funding for HIV Prevention Go To? The Case of
        Condoms Versus Microbicides and Vaccines." *Globalization and Health* 6(23).
        doi:10.1186/1744-8603-6-23.
Petros, George, Collins Airhihenbuwa, Leickness Simbayi,
Shandir Ramlagan, and Brandon Brown
    2006 "HIV/AIDS and 'Othering' in South Africa: The Blame Goes On."
        *Culture, Health & Sexuality* 8(1): 67–77.
Petryna, Adriana
    2005 "Ethical Variability: Drug Development and Globalizing Clinical Trials."
        *American Ethnologist* 32(2): 183–97.

2006  "Globalizing Human Subjects Research." In *Global Pharmaceuticals: Ethics, Markets, Practices*. A. Petryna, A. Lakoff, and A. Kleinman, eds. Pp. 33–63. Durham, NC: Duke University Press.

Pettifor, Audrey, Mags Beksinska, Helen Rees,
Nokuzola Mqoqi, and Kim Dickson-Theti
2001  "The Acceptability of Reuse of the Female Condom among Urban South African Women." *Journal of Urban Health* 78(4): 647–57.

Pettifor, Audrey E., Diana Measham, Helen Rees, and Nancy Padian
2004  "Sexual Power and HIV Risk, South Africa." *Emerging Infectious Diseases* 10(11): 1996–2004.

Phillips, Howard
1990  "The Origin of the Public Health Act of 1919." *South African Medical Journal* 77(10): 531–32.

Pickett, Jim
2013  "VOICE Lesson: It's Unfair to Be Non-Adherent." *IRMA—International Rectal Microbicide Advocates* (blog), 5 March (repost of "VOICE Results Important to New Prevention Technology Research," *HIV Prevention Justice Alliance*, 5 March) *rectalmicrobicides.org*.

Polydex
2007  "Polydex Pharmaceuticals Reports Phase III Trial of Ushercell for HIV Prevention Halted." Press release, 31 January. *marketwired.com*.

Pool, Robert, Catherine M. Montgomery, Neetha S. Morar, Oliver
Mweemba, Agnes Ssali, Mitzy Gafos, Shelley Lees, Jonathan Stadler,
Angela Crook, Andrew Nunn, Richard Hayes, and Sheena McCormack
2010  "A Mixed Methods and Triangulation Model for Increasing the Accuracy of Adherence and Sexual Behaviour Data: The Microbicides Development Programme." *PLoS ONE* 5(7).

Pool, Robert, Khatia Munguambe, Eusebio Macete, Pedro Aide,
Geraldina Juma, Pedro Alonso, and Clara Menendez
2006  "Community Response to Intermittent Preventive Treatment Delivered to Infants (Ipti) through the EPI System in Manhiça, Mozambique." *Tropical Medicine & International Health* 11(11): 1670–78.

Pool, Robert, Stella Nyanzi, and James A. G. Whitworth
2001  "Attitudes to Voluntary Counselling and Testing for HIV among Pregnant Women in Rural South-West Uganda." *AIDS Care* 13(5): 605–15.

Posel, Deborah
2010  "Races to Consume: Revisiting South Africa's History of Race, Consumption and the Struggle for Freedom." *Ethnic and Racial Studies* 33(2): 157–75.

Preda, Alex
    2004   *AIDS, Rhetoric, and Medical Knowledge.* Cambridge: Cambridge University
        Press.
Pronyk, Paul, James P. Hargreaves, Julia C. Kim, Linda A. Morison,
Godfrey Phetla, Charlotte Watts, Joanna Busza, and John D. H. Porter
    2006   "Effect of a Structural Intervention for the Prevention of Intimate-Partner
        Violence and HIV in Rural South Africa: A Cluster Randomised Trial."
        *Lancet* 368(9551): 1937–73.
Ramjee, Gita
    2007   "Commentary 19.1: Ethical Challenges in the N-9 Trial: The Investigator's
        Perspective." In *Ethical Issues in International Biomedical Research: A Casebook.*
        James V. Lavery, Christine Grady, Elizabeth R. Wahl, and Ezekiel J. Emanuel,
        eds. Pp. 314–19. Oxford: Oxford University Press.
Ramjee, Gita, Roshini Govinden, Neetha S. Morar, and Anthony Mbewu
    2007   "South Africa's Experience of the Closure of the Cellulose Sulphate
        Microbicide Trial." *PLoS Medicine* 4(7): e235.
Ramjee, Gita, Anatoli Kamali, and Sheena McCormack
    2010   "The Last Decade of Microbicide Clinical Trials in Africa: From Hypothesis
        to Facts." *AIDS* 24(Supplement 4): S40–49.
Ramjee, Gita, and Salim Abdool Karim
    1998   "Sexually Transmitted Infections among Sex Workers in Kwazulu-Natal,
        South Africa." *Sexually Transmitted Diseases* 25:346–49.
Ramjee, Gita, Neetha S. Morar, Michel Alary, Leonard Mukenge-Tshibaka,
Bea Vuylsteke, Virginie Ettiègne-Traoré, Verapol Chandeying, Salim Abdool
Karim, Lut Van Damme, and on behalf of the COL study group
    2000   "Challenges in the Conduct of Vaginal Microbicide Effectiveness Trials in
        the Developing World." *AIDS* 14(16): 2553–57.
Ramsay, Sarah
    2002   "African Health Researchers Unite." *Lancet* 360:1665–66.
Ravel, Jacques, Pawel Gajer, Li Fu, Christine K. Mauck, Sara S. K. Koenig, Joyce
Sakamoto, Alison A. Motsinger-Reif, Gustavo F. Doncel, and Steven L. Zeichner
    2012   "Twice-Daily Application of HIV Microbicides Alters the Vaginal
        Microbiota." *mBio* 3(6).
Reddy, Priscilla, Dorina Saleh-Onoy, Sibusiso Sifunda, Delia Lang,
Gina Wingood, Bart van den Borne, and Robert A. C. Ruiter
    2009   "Preference for Dry Sex, Condom Use and Risk of STI among HIV-
        Negative Black Women in the Western Cape Province, South Africa." *South
        African Journal of Science* 105(January/February): 73–76.

Reiser, Stanley J.

    1985 "Responsibility for Personal Health: A Historical Perspective." *Journal of Medical Philosophy* 10(1): 7–17.

Roberts, Eric T., and Derrick D. Matthews

    2012 "HIV and Chemoprophylaxis, the Importance of Considering Social Structures alongside Biomedical and Behavioral Intervention." *Social Science & Medicine* 75(9): 1555–61.

Robins, Steven

    2006 "From 'Rights' to 'Ritual": AIDS Activism in South Africa." *American Anthropologist* 108(2): 312–23.

Robinson, Elizabeth T., Deborah Baron, Lori L.

Heise, Jill Moffett, and Sarah V. Harlan

    2010 *Communications Handbook for Clinical Trials: Strategies, Tips, and Tools to Manage Controversy, Convey Your Message, and Disseminate Results.* Research Triangle Park, NC: Family Health International.

Rosenberg, Zeda

    2007 "Statement on the Closing of Cellulose Sulfate Gel Trials due to Concerns of Potential Increased Risk of HIV Infection: International Partnership for Microbicides." International Partnership for Microbicides, 31 January. *ipmglobal.org.*

Runganga, Agnes O., and Jonathan Kasule

    1995 "The Vaginal Use of Herbs/Substances: An HIV Transmission Facilitatory Factor?" *AIDS Care* 7(5): 639–45.

Sabatier, Renée

    1988 *Blaming Others: Prejudice, Race and Worldwide AIDS.* London: Panos Institute.

Saethre, Eirik, and Jonathan Stadler

    2009 "A Tale of Two Cultures: HIV Risk Narratives in South Africa." *Medical Anthropology* 28(3): 1–17.

    2013 "Malicious Whites, Greedy Women, and Virtuous Volunteers: Negotiating Social Relations through Clinical Trial Narratives in South Africa." *Medical Anthropology Quarterly* 27(1): 103–20.

Salyer, David

    2001 "The Scandal of Nonoxynol-9." *The Body*, May. *thebody.com*

Sapire, Hilary

    1992 "Politics and Protest in Shack Settlements of the Pretoria-Witwatersrand-Vereeniging Region, South Africa, 1980–1990." *Journal of Southern African Studies* 18(3): 670–97.

Saxon, Bonnie Jeanne
    2012 "Feasibility of Telephonic Unblinding as Part of a Randomized Controlled Trial Results Dissemination Plan in the South African Context." MPH thesis, University of the Witwatersrand.
Scheper-Hughes, Nancy
    1996 "Theft of Life: The Globalization of Organ Stealing Rumours." *Anthropology Today* 12(3): 3–11.
Scorgie, Fiona, Busisiwe Kunene, Jennifer A. Smit, Ntsiki Manzini,
Matthew F. Chersich, and Eleanor M. Preston-Whyte
    2009 "In Search of Sexual Pleasure and Fidelity: Vaginal Practices in KwaZulu-Natal, South Africa." *Culture, Health & Sexuality* 11(3): 267–83.
Scott, James C.
    1985 *Weapons of the Weak: Everyday Forms of Peasant Resistance.* New Haven, CT: Yale University Press.
Segal, I., and L. O. Tim
    1979 "The Witchdoctor and the Bowel." *South African Medical Journal* 56(8): 308–10.
Shand, Alex
    2005 "Rejoinder: In Defense of Medical Anthropology." *Anthropology & Medicine* 12(2): 105–13.
Shisana, O., T. Rehle, L. C. Simbayi, K. Zuma, S. Jooste,
N. Zungu, D. Labadarios, and D. Onoya
    2014 *South African National HIV Prevalence, Incidence and Behaviour Survey, 2012.* Cape Town: HSRC Press.
Singer, Merrill, and Hans Baer
    1995 *Critical Medical Anthropology.* Amityville, NY: Baywood.
Skafte, Ina, and Margrethe Silberschmidt
    2014 Female Gratification, Sexual Power and Safer Sex: Female Sexuality as an Empowering Resource among Women in Rwanda. *Culture, Health & Sexuality* 16(1): 1–13.
Skoler-Karpoff, Stephanie, Gita Ramjee, Khatija Ahmed, Lydia Altini,
Marlena Gehret Plagianos, Barbara Friedland, Sumen Govender,
Alana De Kock, Nazira Cassim, and Thesla Palanee
    2008 "Efficacy of Carraguard for Prevention of HIV Infection in Women in South Africa: A Randomised, Double-Blind, Placebo-Controlled Trial." *Lancet* 372(9654): 1977–87.
Sobo, Elisa
    1993 "Bodies, Kin, and Flow: Family Planning in Rural Jamaica." *Medical Anthropology Quarterly* 7(1): 50–73.

1995  *Choosing Unsafe Sex: AIDS Risk Denial among Disadvantaged Women.*
Philadelphia: University of Pennsylvania Press.

SOJO Business and Tourism Forum

2016  "Shopping Centers." SOJO Business and Tourism Forum, accessed 10 May.
*sojo.co.za/shopping-centers.aspx.*

Sow, P. S., B. Gueye, O. Sylla, M.A. Faye, and A. M. Coll-Seck

1998  "Pratiques traditionnelles et transmission de l'infection à VIH au Sénégal:
L'exemple du lévirat et du sororat" (Traditional practices and HIV transmission
in Senegal: The example of levirat and sororat). *Médecine et Maladies Infectieuses*
28(2): 203–5.

Spronk, R.

2005  "Female Sexuality in Nairobi: Flawed or Favoured?" *Culture, Health &
Sexuality* 7(3): 267–77.

Stadler, Jonathan

2003  "Rumour, Gossip and Blame: Implications for HIV/AIDS Prevention
in the South African Lowveld." *AIDS Education and Prevention* 15(4):
357–68.

Stadler, Jonathan, C. Dugmore, E. Venables, C. MacPhail, and S. Delany-Moretlwe

2013  "Cognitive Mapping: Using Local Knowledge for Planning Health
Research." *BMC Medical Research Methodologies* 13:96.

Stein, Zena

1990  "HIV Prevention: The Need for Methods Women Can Use." *American
Journal of Public Health* 80:460–62.

Stein, Zena, Landon Myer, and Mervyn Susser

2003  "The Design of Prophylactic Trials for HIV: The Case of Microbicides."
*Epidemiology* 14(1): 80–83.

Stein, Zena, and Ida Susser

2010  "Microbicide Success: New Opportunities for Women" *ALQ/Mujeres
Adelante* (October): 38–42. *www.womeneurope.net/resources/ALQ-Mujeres_
Adelante_October_2010.pdf.*

Stillwaggon, Eileen

2003  "Racial Metaphors: Interpreting Sex and AIDS in Africa." *Development and
Change* 34(5): 809–32.

Stocking, George W.

1982  *Race, Culture, and Evolution: Essays in the History of Anthropology.* Chicago:
University of Chicago Press.

Susser, Ida

2002  "Health Rights for Women in the Age of AIDS." *International Journal of
Epidemiology* 31:45–48.

Tallis, Vicci
    2012 *Feminisms, HIV and AIDS: Subverting Power, Reducing Vulnerability.*
        Hampshire, UK: Palgrave MacMillan.
Tamale, Sylvia
    2011 *African Sexualities: A Reader.* Cape Town: Pambazuka Press.
Tatoud, Roger
    2012 "Disseminating the MDP301 Results: A Critical Approach to the
        Dissemination of Trial Results in a Connected World." Presentation at the
        7th International Microbicides Conference, Sydney, April.
Taylor, Christopher C.
    1990 "Condoms and Cosmology: The 'Fractal' Person and Sexual Risk in
        Rwanda." *Social Science & Medicine* 31:1023–28.
Taylor, Julie J.
    2007 "Assisting or Compromising Intervention? The Concept of 'Culture' in
        Biomedical and Social Research on HIV/AIDS." *Social Science & Medicine*
        64:965–75.
Thege, Britta
    2009 "Rural Black Women's Agency within Intimate Partnerships amid the
        South African HIV Epidemic." *African Journal of AIDS Research* 8(4):
        455–64.
Thom, Anso
    2013 "Africa: Big Prevention Blow as Women Reject One-a-Day ARV." *Health-e
        News* (Cape Town), 4 March. *health-e.org.za.*
Thomas, Keith
    1997 "Health and Morality in Early Modern England." In *Morality and Health.*
        A. M. Brandt and P. Rozin, eds. Pp. 15–33. New York: Routledge.
Thornton, Robert
    2008 *Unimagined Community: Sex, Networks and AIDS in Uganda and South
        Africa.* Berkeley: University of California Press.
Tishler, Carl L., and Suzanne Bartholomae.
    2003 "Repeat Participation among Normal Healthy Research Volunteers:
        Professional Guinea Pigs in Clinical Trials?" *Perspectives in Biology and
        Medicine* 46(4): 508–20.
Tollman, Stephen
    1991 "Community Oriented Primary Care: Origins, Evolution, Applications."
        *Social Science & Medicine* 32(6): 633–42.
Tomes, Nancy
    1997 "Moralizing the Microbe: The Germ Theory and the Moral Construction
        of Behavior in the Late-Nineteenth-Century Antituberculosis Movement. In
        *Morality and Health.* A. M. Brandt and P. Rozin, eds. Pp. 271–96. New York:
        Routledge.

1999 *The Gospel of Germs: Men, Women, and the Microbe in American Life.* Cambridge, MA: Harvard University Press.

Treichler, Paula

1991 "AIDS, Africa, and Cultural Theory." *Transition* 51:86–103.

1999 *How to Have Theory in an Epidemic.* Durham, NC: Duke University Press.

Tsing, Anna

2011 *Friction: An Ethnography of Global Connection.* Princeton, NJ: Princeton University Press.

UNECA (United Nations Economic Commission for Africa)

2008 *Securing Our Future: Report of the Commission on HIV/AIDS and Governance in Africa.* Geneva: UNECA. *uneca.org.*

Vallely, Andrew, Charles Shagi, Stella Kasindi, Nicola Desmond, Shelley Lees, Betty Chiduo, Richard Hayes, Caroline Allen, David Ross, and the Microbicides Development Programme

2007 "The Benefits of Participatory Methodologies to Develop Effective Community Dialogue in the Context of a Microbicide Trial Feasibility Study in Mwanza, Tanzania." *BMC Public Health* 7(133).

Van Damme, Lut

2004 "Clinical Microbicide Research: An Overview." *Tropical Medicine & International Health* 9(12): 1290–96.

Van Damme, Lut, Ann Wright, Katrien Depraetere, Isobel Rosenstein, Veerle Vandersmissen, Len Poulter, Margo McKinlay, Eddy Van Dyck, Jonathan Weber, Al Profy, Marie Laga, and Val Kitchen

2000 "A Phase I Study of a Novel Potential Intravaginal Microbicide, PRO 2000, in Healthy Sexually Inactive Women." *Sexually Transmitted Infections* 76(2): 126–30.

van der Geest, Sjaak

2005 "'Sacraments' in the Hospital: Exploring the Magic and Religion of Recovery." *Anthropology & Medicine* 12(2): 135–50.

van der Geest, Sjaak, and Susan Reynolds Whyte

1989 "The Charm of Medicines: Metaphors and Metonyms." *Medical Anthropology Quarterly* 3(4): 345–67.

van der Straten, Ariane, Elizabeth Montgomery, Diantha Pillay, Helen Cheng, Anushka Naidoo, Zakhele Cele, Kalendri Naidoo, Miriam Hartmann, Jeanna Piper, and Gonasagrie Nair

2013 "Feasibility, Performance, and Acceptability of the Wisebag™ for Potential Monitoring of Daily Gel Applicator Use in Durban, South Africa." *AIDS and Behavior* 17(2): 640–48.

van der Straten, Ariane, Lut Van Damme, Jessica E. Haberer, and David R. Bangsberg

2012 "Unraveling the Divergent Results of Pre-Exposure Prophylaxis Trials for HIV Prevention." *AIDS* 26(7): F13–F19.

van de Wijgert, Janneke H. H. M., Gertrude N. Khumalo-Sakutukwa,
Christiana Coggins, Sabada E. Dube, Prisca Nyamapfeni,
Magdalene Mwale, and Nancy S. Padian
    1999  "Men's Attitudes toward Vaginal Microbicides and Microbicide Trials in
        Zimbabwe." *International Family Planning Perspectives* 25(1): 15–21.
van de Wijgert, Janneke, and Heidi Jones
    2006  "Challenges in Microbicide Trial Design and Implementation." *Studies in
        Family Planning* 37(2): 123–29.
van Dyk, Alta C.
    2001  "Traditional African Beliefs and Customs: Implications for AIDS
        Education and Prevention in Africa." *South Africa Journal of Psychology* 31(2):
        60–67.
Varmus, Harold, and David Satcher
    1997  "Ethical Complexities of Conducting Research in Developing Countries."
        *New England Journal of Medicine* 337(14): 1003–5.
Volpp, Leti
    2000  "Blaming Culture for Bad Behavior." *Yale Journal of Law & Humanities*
        12:89–117.
Wallace, Andrea R., Aaron Teitelbaum, Livia Wan, Maria Gloria Mulima,
Laura Guichard, Stephanie Skiler, Hlengiwe Vilakazi et al.
    2007  "Determining the Feasibility of Utilizing the Microbicide Applicator
        Compliance Assay for Use in Clinical Trials." *Contraception* 76:53–56.
Weber, Jonathan, Kamal Desai, Janet Darbyshire on
behalf of the Microbicides Development Programme
    2005  "The Development of Vaginal Microbicides for the Prevention of HIV
        Transmission." *PLoS Med* 2(5): e142.
Weiss, Helen A., Daniel Halperin, Robert C. Bailey,
Richard J. Hayes, George Schmid, and Catherine A. Hankins
    2008  "Male Circumcision for HIV Prevention: From Evidence to Action?"
        *AIDS* 22(5): 567–74.
Westercamp, Nelli, and R. C. Bailey
    2007  "Acceptability of Male Circumcision for Prevention of HIV/AIDS in Sub-
        Saharan Africa: A Review." *AIDS and Behavior* 11(3): 341–55.
White, Charles
    1799  *An Account of the Regular Gradation in Man.* London: C. Dilly.
White, Luise
    2000  *Speaking with Vampires: Rumor and History in Colonial Africa.* Berkeley:
        University of California Press.
WHO (World Health Organization)
    2010  *Preparing for Access to PRO 2000 Microbicide.* Geneva: World Health
        Organization.

Whyte, Susan Reynolds, Sjaak van der Geest, and Anita Hardon
  2002  *The Social Lives of Medicines*. Cambridge: Cambridge University Press.
Whyte, Susan Reynolds, Michael A. Whyte, Lotte Meinert, and Betty Kyaddondo
  2006  "Treating AIDS: Dilemmas of Unequal Access in Uganda." In *Global
    Pharmaceuticals: Ethics, Markets, Practices*. A. Petryna, A. Lakoff, and A.
    Kleinman, eds. Pp. 240–64. Durham, NC: Duke University Press.
Wilcox, Allen
  2003  "Voices: A Conversation with Zena Stein." *Epidemiology* 14:498–502.
Wilkinson, David
  2002a  "Condom Effectiveness in Reducing Heterosexual HIV Transmission."
    *WHO Reproductive Health Library*, 11 November.
  2002b  "Nonoxynol-9 Fails to Prevent STDs, But Microbicide Research
    Continues." *Lancet* 360(9338): 962–63.
Wilkinson, David, Maya Tholandi, Gita Ramjee, and George W. Rutherford
  2002  "Nonoxynol-9 Spermicide for Prevention of Vaginally Acquired HIV and
    Other Sexually Transmitted Infections: Systematic Review and Meta-Analysis
    of Randomised Controlled Trials Including More than 5000 Women." *Lancet
    Infectious Diseases* 2(10): 613–17.
Winslow, Charles-Edward Amory
  1920  "The Untilled Fields of Public Health." *Science* 51(1306): 23–33.
Wojcicki, Janet
  2002a  "Commercial Sex Work or Ukuphanda? Sex for Money Exchange in
    Soweto and Hamanskraal Area." *Culture, Medicine and Psychiatry* 26(3):
    339–70.
  2002b  "'She Drank His Money': Survival Sex and the Problem of Violence in
    Taverns in Gauteng South Africa." *Medical Anthropology Quarterly* 16(3):
    1–28.
Wojcicki, Janet, and Josephine Malala
  2001  "Condom Use, Power and HIV/AIDS Risk: Sex-Workers Bargain for
    Survival in Hillbrow/Joubert Park/Berea, Johannesburg." *Social Science &
    Medicine* 53:99–121.
Wood, Katherine, and Rachel Jewkes
  2006  "Blood Blockages and Scolding Nurses: Barriers to Adolescent
    Contraceptive Use in South Africa." *Reproductive Health Matters* 14:109–18.
Wood, Katherine, Fidelia Maforah, and Rachel Jewkes
  1998  "'He Forced Me to Love Him': Putting Violence on Adolescent Sexual
    Health Agendas." *Social Science & Medicine* 47(2): 233–42.
Woodsong, Cynthia, Kathleen MacQueen, K. Rivet Amico, Barbara Friedland,
Mitzy Gafos, Leila Mansoor, Elizabeth Tolley, and Sheena McCormack
  2013  "Microbicide Clinical Trial Adherence: Insights for Introduction." *Journal
    of the International AIDS Society* 16(18505): 1–9.

Worboys, Michael
    1990  "Manson, Ross and Colonial Medical Policy: Tropical Medicine in London
        and Liverpool, 1899–1914." In *Disease, Medicine and Empire: Perspectives on
        Western Medicine and the Experience of European Expansion*. R. Macleod and
        M. Lewis, eds. Pp. 21–37. New York: Routledge.
Yamba, C. Bawa
    1997  "Cosmologies in Turmoil: Witchfinding and AIDS in Chiawa, Zambia."
        *Africa* 67(2): 200–23.
Yoshioka, Alan
    1998  "Use of Randomisation in the Medical Research Council's Clinical Trial
        of Streptomycin in Pulmonary Tuberculosis in the 1940s." *British Medical
        Journal* 317:1220–23.
Youssef, H.
    1993  "The History of the Condom." *Journal of the Royal Society of Medicine*
        86:226–28.

# Index